"Going vegan has always been about love for all life, and this book shows that it's just what the doctor—and his champion athlete coauthor—ordered for your love life too."

Victoria Moran
AUTHOR OF *MAIN STREET VEGAN*

"The only thing better than a good morning is a wood morning! ED has been called ground zero of cardiovascular disease. A morning erection can serve as a daily systems check that should put a smile on your face . . . and maybe even your partner's."

Marco Borges
AUTHOR OF *THE 22 DAYS REVOLUTION*

"This book will instruct you how to improve blood vessel function and return to the nature we were meant to have. Let's change our lifestyles and really enjoy our lives."

Kim A. William Sr., MD
CARDIOLOGIST, RUSH UNIVERSITY MEDICAL CENTER

"The same diet that closes the arteries to the heart and brain has the same effect on other arteries—and often arterial function decline shows up first in organs other than the heart. Isn't it time we bring this behind-closed-doors conversation out into the light of day?"

Lani Muelrath
AUTHOR OF *THE PLANT-BASED JOURNEY, FIT QUICKIES, THE MINDFUL VEGAN*

"Healthy eating can add more than just years to your life—it can add life to your years. Healthy people have more fun! Read this book to learn how."

Michael Greger, MD
AUTHOR OF *HOW NOT TO DIE*

"Proven by research studies and personal experience, and written in an engaging—sometimes irreverent—style, this simple method works better than a wheelbarrow full of Viagra."

Neal D. Barnard, MD
PRESIDENT, PHYSICIANS COMMITTEE

about the authors

ELLEN JAFFE JONES is an inspiring motivational speaker, certified personal trainer, running coach, author, and a cooking class instructor for the Physicians Committee for Responsible Medicine (PCRM). She was an award-winning TV investigative reporter and anchor in Miami and St. Louis, and then became a successful financial consultant specializing in socially responsible and animal-friendly investments at Smith Barney.

Ellen is a champion runner in both endurance and sprint events, a rare accomplishment. She is currently a nationally ranked sprinter, coming in third and fifth in races in the women's 65 to 69 age group, and has placed in over 130 races that are 5K or longer, including four senior grand masters. For more information, visit vegcoach.com.

JOEL K. KAHN, MD, is a clinical professor of medicine at Wayne State University School of Medicine and a summa cum laude graduate of the University of Michigan School of Medicine. He lectures widely on the benefits of nutrition for cardiac health, mind-body practices, and heart attack prevention. Dr. Kahn founded the Kahn Center for Cardiac Longevity and owns GreenSpace Cafe in Detroit. For more information, visit drjoelkahn.com.

BEVERLY LYNN BENNETT is an experienced vegan chef and baker, writer, and animal advocate who is passionate about showing the world how easy, delicious, and healthy it is to live and eat as a vegan. A certified food-service operations manager, she earned her culinary arts degree in 1988 from the University of Akron, Ohio, and in the following years worked in and managed vegan and vegetarian restaurants and natural food stores.

Beverly currently lives and works in Eugene, Oregon, where her love of organic, healthy, and vibrant foods fuels a passion for developing innovative vegan recipes. For more information, visit veganchef.com.

REVISED

vegan SEX

DUMP YOUR MEDS AND JUMP IN BED

ellen jaffe jones

AND

joel k. kahn, MD

RECIPES BY

beverly lynn bennett

Healthy Living Publications

SUMMERTOWN, TENNESSEE

Library of Congress Cataloging-in-Publication Data

Names: Jones, Ellen Jaffe, author. | Kahn, Joel K., author.
Title: Vegan sex revised : dump your meds and jump in bed / Ellen Jaffe Jones and Joel K. Kahn, MD ; recipes by Beverly Lynn Bennett.
Other titles: Vegan sex
Description: Summertown, TN : Healthy Living Publications, 2018. | Revision of: Vegan sex. 2017. First edition. | Includes bibliographical references and index.
Identifiers: LCCN 2018004359 (print) | LCCN 2018005447 (ebook) | ISBN 9781570678455 (E-book) | ISBN 9781570673610 (pbk.)
Subjects: LCSH: Sexual health. | Veganism.
Classification: LCC RA788 (ebook) | LCC RA788 .J678 2018 (print) | DDC 613.9/6—dc23
LC record available at https://lccn.loc.gov/2018004359

Nutrition Breakdowns for Recipes: The nutrient values provided for the recipes in this book are estimates only, calculated from the individual ingredients used in each recipe based on the nutrition data found for those ingredients. Optional items are not included. Nutrient content may vary based on methods of preparation, origin and freshness of ingredients, product brands, and other factors.

We chose to print this title on sustainably harvested paper stock certified by the Forest Stewardship Council, an independent auditor of responsible forestry practices. For more information, visit https://us.fsc.org.

FSC
www.fsc.org
MIX
Paper from responsible sources
FSC® C005010

Cover and interior design: John Wincek
Stock photography: 123 RF

Printed in the United States of America

Healthy Living Publications
A division of Book Publishing Company
PO Box 99
Summertown, TN 38483
888-260-8458
bookpubco.com

Disclaimer: The information in this book is presented for educational purposes only. It isn't intended to be a substitute for the medical advice of a physician, dietitian, or other health-care professional.

ISBN: 978-1-57067-361-0

23 22 21 20 19 18 1 2 3 4 5 6 7 8 9

contents

dedication

To my daughters, Rebecca, Jessica, and Aron. Our children's future prospects for a healthy life and planet depend on whether we get global warming, climate change, and both human and non-human health right as soon as possible.

To Bob and Cynthia Holzapfel, who said yes to my very first book and haven't wavered since. Their partnership is a behind-the-scenes force in the vegan universe. They've given the world some of the first widely read and distributed vegan books and support the voices of so many of us who are trying to speak for those who can't speak on their own behalf.

And to my parents, who were so sick and diseased they couldn't lift my babies, let alone babysit them. Entire generations are losing each other and don't even know it. Preventable pain and suffering should not exist anywhere, not in this day and age.

Ellen Jaffe Jones

acknowledgments

So many people contributed to this book, knowingly or not. First, I need to thank the amazing Joel Kahn, MD, otherwise humbly known on social media and elsewhere as " America's Healthy Heart Doc." We were both speakers at a South Florida Vegfest one year, and when I saw his "Vegan Is Sexy" T-shirt, I said half joking, "Ya know, I'm writing a book called *Vegan Sex*. Want to coauthor it?" Dr. Kahn immediately and kindly said yes. He shared my belief and vision, and I was especially excited to have a cardiologist on board.

A big thanks to superstar recipe developer and author Beverly Lynn Bennett. You're going to love her contributions—plus, she's been loving and having fabulous sex with the same vegan guy for over thirty years.

Others contributed to this book with their stories, experience, and knowledge. I opted to keep some of them anonymous, as it was very painful for them to share their narratives. I appreciate their courage and candor. You know who you are. The list of those OK with being acknowledged includes but isn't limited to Reggie Adams, Steve Blumberg, Trevor Chin, Rebecca Gilbert, Bob and Cynthia Holzapfel, David Kidd, Gabrielle Lennon, Jack McMillan, Alan Roettinger, Miyoko Schinner, everyone in Florida Voices for Animals, and animal and vegan activists everywhere—plus a slew of unnamed ex-boyfriends and partners who were part of failed relationships. Failure can be our greatest teacher.

There are courageous vegan doctors and dietitians who have risked their reputations and livelihoods to go against the ways of conventional medicine and truly do no harm. They should all win Nobel prizes for following their consciences and doing what's in the best interests of patients and clients.

A special thanks to my dear friend Jen Kaden, who's done so much to help organize the Cleveland Vegfest, one of the best and biggest vegan gatherings in the United States. Her organizational and interpersonal skills are extraordinary, and she's been a great mentor.

Finally, thanks to my special friend Val McDaniel, one of the most thoughtful and giving people I've ever met. He regularly asks, "What can I do today to make you happy?" and performs many random acts of kindness for me. I wasn't used to that type of generosity and didn't think it was possible of anyone in this very cranky, mixed-up world. He keeps me motivated and focused on the toughest of days. He noticed all kinds of changes, both in and out of bed, as he became vegan. Watching his transformation as he transitioned from smoking and eating steak to exercising and eating healthy was one of the main inspirations for this book. I fully realized the impact of his change when his daughter gave him a handmade shirt with the question "What happens when you eat vegan?" on the front. The underside of the shirt reads: "She moans." I'll let you interpret that however you like. Val's editing skills were invaluable, and he also provided many yucks for my coauthors and me by googling "vegetables that look like sex organs." We had no idea! We'll never look at oranges and radishes the same way again.

Warning! This is somewhat of an X-rated book. By definition, it has to be. I mean, you can't really talk about sex without, well, talking about sex. Realizing how great vegan sex is for you, your partner, the planet, and the animals will lift your spirits. If you find yourself shocked or even outraged at the differences between vegan and nonvegan sex, you may wonder, as I did, why did it take so long to find out?

Ellen Jaffe Jones

1 what is vegan sex?

by Ellen Jaffe Jones

Is healthy sex that important? Yes, absolutely! Who knows how many marriages might have been saved if there had been great sex to spice up the tedium that can set in over time or relieve the anxiety simply from living in a crazy-and-getting-crazier world.

I know sex isn't everything. Although having an OK body can stimulate attraction and interest, I always wanted the focus to be on my heart and brains—something other than just my looks. I also wanted to like my partners for their kindness, compassion, empathy, smarts, and big hearts, and I hoped it would work the same way in return. But, as I would learn, physical attraction and emotional intimacy can go a long way to bridge the chasms, disagreements, and differences between lovers. And even more, the heart–mind connection is intricately interwoven in the expression of sexuality. That's the 95 percent of sex that happens between the ears.

WHAT IT MEANS TO BE VEGAN

Before we can talk about vegan sex, we need to talk about what it means to be a vegan. Basically, vegans don't eat, use, buy, or exploit anything with a mother or a face. So no consumption of meat or animal products at all. No eggs, no dairy, no honey. (Yes, taking honey from hives does stress bees. Maybe you've heard it's good for them, but it isn't.)

The thought of giving up favorite comfort foods can be dismaying. Because people who switch to a vegan diet are no longer getting protein from familiar animal foods, their greatest fear is developing a severe protein deficiency. The truth is, the largest, studliest animals on the planet are plant eaters. Think bison, elephants, giraffes, hippopotamuses, horses, manatees, rhinoceroses, some whales, wildebeest, and yaks. All are magnificent, powerful, and definitely not lacking in protein or energy. If they can thrive on plants, so can humans, and we now have scientific evidence that proves just that. It might surprise you to know that almost all plant foods have a certain amount of protein—even a banana has one gram! Bottom line, it's tough to eat all the calories you need from a variety of plant foods and *not* get enough protein.

People are motivated to become vegan for a variety of reasons. My journey to veganism actually began as a five-year-old when my aunt died of breast cancer. I subsequently watched my mom and both sisters get breast cancer, as well as various combinations of heart disease, diabetes, diverticulitis, Alzheimer's, arthritis, macular degeneration, and varicose veins—so many of the diseases of affluence that are perpetuated by a diet full of meat and dairy products.

At the age of twenty-eight, I collapsed and almost died of a colon blockage. The first thing I did to prevent a recurrence was read five books about fiber—that was the sum total of all the books on fiber available at that time. The research and writings by surgeon and fiber expert Denis Burkitt really opened my eyes. I realized that in some places of the world, mainly Africa, where primitive high-fiber diets were commonplace, people had bowel movements as frequently as three times a day. In my world, having three movements a week was cause for celebration. I began adding loose bran fiber to my cereals and was blown away by how effective that simple change was. I got even more positive results by switching to a diet rich in vegetables, fruits, and whole grains.

My attempts to eat a clean diet went in fits and starts until I did an investigative piece on animal cruelty as a local TV journalist in Miami. I scoped out how animals from the Miami city animal shelter were not properly euthanized before being disposed of at the city dump. The similarities between that situation and how cruelly animals are butchered at processing plants helped me connect the dots between diet and compassion.

Then I heard Neal Barnard, MD, president of the Physicians Committee for Responsible Medicine (PCRM), speak in my hometown of St. Louis. His message linking a vegan diet to optimal health resonated deeply with me because I'd spent a lifetime in hospitals watching so many of my family members struggle with—and sometimes die of—diet-related diseases. As the very youngest in my family, I had many years to see what didn't work and how I didn't want to live my life. I knew there must be a better way. I would soon learn that most of my relatives' illnesses were totally preventable. At that point I was well on my way to becoming a staunch advocate for the positive impact a vegan diet would have for the animals, the environment, and people's health.

VEGAN SEX AND ERECTILE DYSFUNCTION

What makes sex vegan? If you've made love to a vegan, you've had vegan sex. If you haven't, you're a vegan virgin. I had never had sex with a vegan until I was in my sixties. When I did, it blew my mind. I've had sexual experiences with both vegans and nonvegans and the contrast was stark. Above all, I was elated not to face issues of deflation, so to speak, and by that I'm talking about erectile dysfunction.

Erectile dysfunction (ED) is defined as the inability of the male penis to maintain an erection. Its principal cause, artery disease, can be the elephant in the bedroom. By and large, ED is all about lack of blood flow. Normally an erect penis contains up to eight times the amount of blood it has when it's flaccid, but clogged arteries may create a work stoppage—or a downright strike. Even worse, the presence of ED can indicate serious health problems. My coauthor, cardiologist Joel Kahn, will share with you a detailed medical description of this condition in chapters 2 and 3.

Although people should be worried about the serious health implications that ED points to, the fact is, they're more likely to be hurt and disappointed with how it contributes to a lack of intimacy in the bedroom. Both sexes can be left with feelings of dissatisfaction, inadequacy, and emotional loss that will seriously affect their relationships. Becoming vegan can actually improve ED by reversing artery disease. This book will tell you how and why.

I love this testimonial, a personal story from a recently converted vegan, now sexually active, who had given up on sex for decades: "After a man fails two or three times in a row, he starts to believe he'll never have an erection again. It becomes a self-fulfilling prophecy that's very difficult to stop. This feeling of inadequacy is what the drug companies feed on to sell their ED drugs. If you go vegan and get off the drugs, you won't need to build two side-by-side bathtubs outside, as shown in one of the prevalent ads, or anywhere. Hanging out in one tub, inside, will be just dandy and all you'll ever need for those magical moments."

Got Viagra?

You've probably heard the warning that's aired at the end of commercials about ED drugs: "If you have an erection lasting more than four hours, call your doctor." Or as some of my vegan women friends now say, "Forget the doctor. Call me!"

Here are the words of a man recovering from ED who hasn't taken Viagra in nearly a year after switching to an almost totally vegan diet: "ED lowers people's spirits. They feel less capable. They become less active. They feel less desirable to potential partners. They retreat into believing they're just getting old. The downward spiral begins, and the rest of their health follows downward also."

I know that a vegan diet isn't a guaranteed buffer against all diseases and conditions. When I first came up with the concept for this book, some of my vegan women friends adamantly responded: "Nope, not so fast. My husband is vegan and has erectile dysfunction." However, from my research and personal experience, I believe that the odds of not having ED are much better for vegans. And if they do have ED, they have a better chance of achieving at least a partial erection. A little bit can go a long way.

BEING VEGAN MAKES FOR BETTER SEX

Vegans do it better because, broadly speaking, they're generally in better physical shape than nonvegans. Studies show that vegans' hearts are more fully functional and their body weights are lower than nonvegans. This allows more vegans to readily participate in sports or fitness activities that help them achieve and maintain their physical prowess. A wholesome, balanced vegan diet, rich in antioxidants and phytochemicals, is also well known for increasing vitality on the inside and outside. Not surprisingly, vegans often look younger than their years. The stamina that allows them to be in great shape out of bed transfers directly to the bedroom. If you've ever had sex with a long-time smoker who's starting to develop emphysema, you're no doubt aware when stamina diminishes. It's difficult for people with this type of health condition to breathe, and in some cases, it's impossible for them to reach orgasm because they can't breathe deeply enough to reach the finish line.

In addition to better stamina, there are other reasons why vegans have an advantage in terms of sexual energy, enjoyment, and performance:

A Video Is Worth a Thousand Words

Vegan doctors are working hard to get the message across. Terry Mason, MD, chief operating officer at the Chicago Department of Public Health, has been a urological surgeon for thirty years. He shows incredibly graphic videos of penile implant surgeries while on the lecture circuit. He concludes his presentations (which, trust me, you'll never forget) by saying, "All men ought to be required to watch this. If they knew what was in store for them as a result of eating an artery-clogging diet, they would change their diets to plant-based in a heartbeat!"

BETTER VASCULAR HEALTH. Contrary to conventional wisdom, ED isn't caused by anxiety. More often it's the result of physical and sometimes psychological problems. The biggest obstacle to a hard penis is blood flow. Studies have found that up to 75 percent of heart disease patients have ED. The saturated fat in meat restricts blood flow throughout the body, making it difficult for enough blood to not only find its way into the penis but also into the vagina, labia, and clitoris. (Yes, even the clitoris needs to get blood flow in order to rise to the occasion.) A diet that includes meat and dairy products can cause an increase in blood pressure, requiring medications that restrict blood flow and can also lead to ED.

DEEPER DESIRE. Some foods cause a chemical reaction in the body that increases libido in both males and females. Foods with large amounts of B vitamins and zinc are believed to elevate testosterone levels and boost sexual desire. Some health professionals are concerned that vegans will have low zinc levels, but foods that supply zinc can be found throughout the plant kingdom. Common plant foods that are rich in B vitamins as well as zinc include almonds, asparagus, avocados, bananas, basil, cashews, celery, chickpeas, figs, kidney beans, pine nuts, and pumpkin seeds. See chapter 7 for information about these foods.

MORE PLANTS, MORE SEMEN. The reason for this is that semen contains vitamin C and zinc, two nutrients that are abundant in plant foods. For example, citrus fruits are high in vitamin C, and Brazil nuts, cashews, flaxseeds, kidney beans, pumpkin seeds, and spinach are rich in zinc.

EXTRA MOISTURE. If your body is getting all the water it needs, it becomes an effervescent production plant of delightful bodily fluids. Translation: You're well lubricated. Losing your natural lubrication as you age doesn't have to be inevitable; eating vegan foods can actually increase it. Foods that have a high water content (especially cantaloupe, cucumbers, and watermelon) help moisturize the skin, but if you pair them with nuts and seeds that contain omega-3 fatty acids (think walnuts and chia, flax, and hemp seeds), you'll have a potent combination for alleviating vaginal dryness. While alcohol and caffeine may increase sex drive by removing barriers and inhibitions, they're also dehydrating. So keep that in mind if vaginal dryness is an issue.

INCREASED HAPPINESS. One study measured the effects of diet and exercise with the effects of meditation. The group that meditated had half the risk of heart attack, stroke, and death than the diet and exercise group. There are a number of studies that found that focusing on compassion lowers heart rate and improves overall well-being. A study done in Australia measured the brain waves of novice and expert meditators who were exposed to both emotional and neutral sounds during meditation. The results showed that concern for others is cultivated during meditation, especially when it's practiced on a regular basis, and helps people become more responsive to sounds of distress. It's widely thought that humans evolved to think more negatively so they would be more easily scared by the presence of wild animals and would therefore be less likely to be eaten by them. Taking pleasure in knowing that you're vegan and not eating any animals (or being chased by wild ones) will help thwart any inclination to revert to the dark side.

SMOOTHER SKIN. A vegan diet rich in life-giving fruits and vegetables, with all their lush antioxidants, has long been praised for giving skin a healthy glow. If your skin feels good, you'll feel good, and you'll have more confidence about your appearance. The hormones contained in fat-laden dairy and animal products store pesticides and other toxins very efficiently and eventually ooze their way to the skin, the largest organ in the body. You may be familiar with toxic outbreaks, such as acne and eczema and itching in places where the sun don't shine.

Consuming plenty of water and water-filled fruits and vegetables also helps to support a glow that radiates from within. So if you're consuming a good amount of these, your body will naturally fight off the chronic dehydration that tends to increase as you age. Also, the vitamin C and antioxidants you'll get from all those plant foods will help your skin wrinkle less and become softer, smoother, and silkier to the touch.

A TASTIER, SWEETER-SMELLING BODY. If you eat more fruit—especially bananas, papayas, and pineapples—bodily fluids will taste sweeter.

Even the chlorophyll in green plants, such as celery and parsley, sweetens the load. Red meat makes semen taste salty. Bitterness in seminal fluid is associated with caffeine, cigarettes, and the preservatives found in processed foods. Some websites say that ejaculate should normally smell like ammonia or chlorine. Maybe that's business as usual for meat eaters, but that's not the experience vegans report. The simple cure for foul-smelling secretions is to eat beautifully aromatic and colorful plants.

Vegans don't get off the hook completely. Vegetables from the sulfur-rich allium and cruciferous families can make semen taste a little like rotten eggs. Allium vegetables include garlic and onions. Cruciferous vegetables include broccoli, kale, and the potentially more-offending cabbage. But don't let the aroma of these nutrient-rich, antioxidant powerhouses scare you from enjoying their many benefits. Garlic, in particular, is associated with increased blood flow. According to anecdotal reports, the semen and body odor of meat eaters is far worse than those of a vegan who just had a bowl of coleslaw.

Eggs create far more offensive body odors than any of these vegetables. Although you might think that eggs would make the body smell like sulfur (the scent of rotten eggs), professionals suggest that rotting fish is more commonly the telltale smell of decomposing eggs in the body. More accurately, it's the breakdown of animal protein and fats that produces flatulence that smells like rotten eggs—which not only is stinky but may also be a sign of colon cancer. If you're already vegan, you know that the smell of your bowel movements prior to your becoming vegan and the smell of your bowel movements now is like night and day. The same applies to body odor, ejaculate, and vaginal fluids.

Check out the "smell study" Dr. Kahn mentions on page 24 that compared the smells from the armpits of meat eaters to those of vegetarians. The veggie group won hands down. The women in the study reported that the meat-eating men really did smell putrid. This corresponds with an experience of a friend of mine who served in the Vietnam war. He was warned by the South Vietnamese that soldiers from the North could smell the Americans before they saw them because of their strong body odor.

SNORING AND SEX

Although sex often takes place before partners go to sleep and snoring occurs after they go to sleep, snoring can exacerbate

A Word about Gender Designations

For the sake of simplicity, I write from my own experience of being female and dealing with men in heterosexual relationships, as that's my orientation. I've never had sex with a woman, so I can't really compare same-sex vegan sex to nonvegan sex except from the interviews I've done. Because I've experienced different men, vegan and not, I can offer my observations of the differences from my perspective.

What I write about, then, reflects my firsthand account of the very obvious changes in men after their adoption of a vegan diet. Different women desire different things in their relationships. While I suspect my experiences aren't uncommon, I can only write from my observations and personal bias. But the genders as I refer to them in this book can be reversed, interchanged, or the same. However it works best for your situation and orientation is all good.

I developed a survey that I gave to a number of people who contributed their ideas to this book. I wanted very much to address some of the main issues facing the LGBTQ community, but I was unable to find anyone willing to answer the survey questions or contribute to the text. Maybe in the next edition.

problems with intimacy and may correlate with erectile dysfunction. Why do people snore? Snoring begins when the nose and throat partially close while a person is prone. Everyone's neck muscles relax during sleep, but if the upper airway is smaller than usual, it vibrates, making the noises we associate with snoring. Snoring can be caused by alcohol consumption, allergies, muscle relaxants, nasal obstruction, and smoking. But the biggest contributor to snoring is obesity. Excess fat doesn't only accumulate in the midsection; it can also build up on the inside of the throat, causing constriction. If obesity is the cause of someone's snoring, vascular health is reduced and ED may also be a problem.

If snoring becomes so loud and incessant that it disrupts the sleep of a partner, the offending person is often banished to a "snore room," an extra room that's distant enough that the non-snoring partner can get a good night's sleep. The time spent sleeping apart can add to a lack of intimacy. But a snore room may also provide an excuse for someone with ED to retreat from the bedroom to avoid another failed sexual experience. If this becomes chronic, sex will fall off the radar completely.

Is snoring part of the aging process? In some cases, perhaps. But I've been so astounded by observations of my older vegan partners. They've been, as many vegans are, at a healthy weight and were quiet as lambs when it came to snoring. Nothing interfered with their sexual performance either, so I'm guessing they had no excess fat clogging their arteries, veins, or throats. Chalk up one more benefit to vegan sex!

THE BENEFITS OF HAVING A VEGAN PARTNER

I want to give a shout-out to vegans everywhere who now travel on this path because they had been curious and willing to get the facts, watched movies and videos, read books, and became involved in their own vegan communities. They should be celebrated and appreciated as role models. These individuals are compassionate and giving in all aspects of their lives. Many volunteer at their local VegFests or animal sanctuaries, take in strays, build cat shelters, or assume leadership roles in animal rights groups or online forums. They may plan meetups and do some of the heavy lifting needed to organize community events. There's not a mean bone in their bodies. They are often fabulous chefs because they've read the same cookbooks as their partners—or at least they've watched their partners cook or have helped with the prep. Some even do all the cleanup, uttering that wonderful phrase, "It's the least I can do." If your dining partner helps you scratch cleanup duty off your to-do list, you'll no doubt want them as a friend for life!

Some people have become vegan because of their partners, and some did it all on their own. Even if men were encouraged to adopt veganism because of their significant other, their ability to stick with it should be appreciated no matter how or why it happened. But since more women are vegan than men, it would be great if more men would take the ball (and their balls) and run with it.

My mission with this book is to let you know how easy and fun it is to live as a vegan—both in and out of bed. This is based on science as well as a lifetime of experience. My motivation, as might be obvious by now, is a bit—well, OK, completely—selfish. I want the world teeming with more vegan men! It's really just that simple. And if you're lucky enough to find a partner who gets it and gets you, count your blessings every day. If not, you might find some interesting tools in these pages to begin your recruitment today. Knowledge is power.

2

of hard attacks and heart attacks

WHY CARDIOLOGISTS SHOULD CARE

by Joel Kahn, MD

Why should a cardiologist care about the quality of your erection? Your ejaculation? Your orgasm? Is it appropriate for a university professor to write about topics usually kept under wraps? Actually, the history and science of sex have been intertwined with heart and artery health for decades. And although not all sex is driven by the emotion of love, the heart as a symbol of love is a clear allegorical union of the pillow and the pump.

Take, for example, the pill that changed male behavior forever. While you might be thinking the birth control pill (which did have a profound impact on increasing sexual activity), I'm referring to the blue pill known as Viagra. Viagra, or sildenafil citrate, wasn't originally intended to make men better in the sack. It was identified as a compound that had favorable effects on arteries and was tested by the giant pharmaceutical house Pfizer for the treatment of high blood pressure and heart disease. One of the most memorable side effects reported by the study participants helped write a new chapter on sex. While the patients in these early trials reported some improvement in cardiac function, they also testified to tighter pants, easier erections, and greater success in completing the sex act. Remember, these were men with cardiovascular disease, and for many of them this was the first time in a long while that the fire below was hot enough to raise the flag pole. They were ecstatic about continuing the drug.

Pfizer sensed they had a winner—just not the one they expected—and shifted the trials to sexual success. The approval process for the drug now known as Viagra proceeded. It was approved by the FDA in 1998 and launched a multibillion-dollar industry. Viagra was recently studied in Sweden, and the results were presented at a national cardiology meeting in 2017. In 43,000 men who had suffered a first heart attack, the use of any erectile dysfunction drugs, including Viagra, Cialis, and Levitra, was observed to reduce the risk of dying of any cause by 33 percent during the course of the three-year study. That's a big advantage to the survivor of a heart attack. It's also gratifying to know the safety of sex in general and these drugs in particular. Surely further research is needed. For now, however, it appears that more blood to the wood is good for the heart and soul.

Why would a drug that's good for heart's arteries prove to be good for the wood too? Is there a link between the sexual response of men and women and cardiovascular health? Actually, there's a very strong connection between arteries and sex organs, as all sex organs (a very dry term for your junk) are supplied by arteries. Taking care of your heart and arteries may be the best sex aid ever. Almost four hundred years ago, English physician Thomas Sydenham wrote that "a man is as old as his arteries." The modern version would be "men, women, and transgender people are as old as their arteries," or as I like to spin it positively, "you are as young as your arteries." Put one more way, "you are as hard as your arteries are soft." My cardiology practice is dedicated to helping arteries stay young for health and longevity.

Every day I ask all my male patients about their ability to develop and maintain an erection. Although the usual response is "strong like bull," many men do have serious problems. Can erectile dysfunction develop as a sign of sick arteries before a life-threatening heart attack or stroke? Yes, and this is *so* important to know: Seek a full evaluation if your penis is not responding like it used to. While I'm certain this is true for women too, there's not much data on female sexual response and heart disease, so forgive me for the male focus in this discussion. Recent data indicate that identifying a man with diabetes who is unable to have a satisfactory erection can predict the presence of diseased arteries and future heart events several years before a heart attack or heart death. The predictive power of erectile dysfunction on heart events is even more powerful than smoking, high blood pressure, or even a family history of early heart attacks.

If you have erectile dysfunction, or sleep with a man who does, getting to the doctor for a complete evaluation may allow time to identify, treat, and reverse arterial damage before bad things happen. Do yourself or your man a favor and share this information in a supportive way. Teaching more people about the data indicating that there is "survival of the firmest" could save many lives. All you have to do is practice a lifestyle that promotes arterial health head to toe, with emphasis on the joy of the groin. Let's learn a bit more about the link between the groin and heart.

THE CONNECTION BETWEEN HEALTHY ARTERIES AND SUCCESSFUL SEX

There are fifty thousand miles of arteries coursing through your body, although guys are mainly concerned with about six inches, not miles. Inside every artery is an inner lining that's only one cell-layer thick called the endothelium. An appreciation of the role of the endothelium for health was so significant that three researchers were awarded the Nobel Prize in Medicine in 1998 for this finding. They figured out that when the endothelium is healthy, it produces a gas called nitric oxide (NO). This is different from nitrous oxide, known as laughing gas. Arteries can make a lot of NO or just a little. When a lot of NO is produced, arteries relax, allowing more blood flow and more normal blood pressure, which decreases the formation of arterial plaque and the blood clots that cause heart attack and stroke. It turns out that to have a great sexual response, lots of NO needs to be present, so lots of blood can be brought in to swell the necessary tissues. Endothelial dysfunction (ED), or "dicksfunction," if you want to make people laugh, leads to a poor blood flow response throughout the body and poor maintenance of the swollen penis needed to create and sustain an erection. Just say yes to NO.

WHAT HARMS YOUR ENDOTHELIUM?

How many times have you heard that eating fruits and vegetables can improve your health? Do you do it? If you do, you are part of the 1.5 percent of Americans who actually practice what I preach regarding healthy eating. If you include the healthy habits of eating well, not smoking, exercising regularly, and maintaining a proper weight, you're among the 3 percent of Americans who go four for four. These are the very lifestyle factors that are known to help the endothelium and its production of NO. Do you like to smoke? You'll make less NO. Do you like to sit and watch movies? You'll make less NO. Do you like to eat fast food and gain weight? You'll make less NO. Do you like donuts more than grapes? You'll make less NO. Lifestyle decisions can lead to diabetes, elevated cholesterol, hypertension, and obesity, and all of these conditions can produce erectile and endothelial dysfunction by the production of less NO.

The standard American diet is high in processed foods packed with chemicals, fat, sugar, and salt and is often combined with a sedentary lifestyle, poorly managed stress, intake of environmental toxins, such as bisphenol A (BPA) found in plastic bottles, and poor sleep. These are all factors that reduce NO and produce ED. Diets emphasizing plant-powered, rainbow-colored foods that are naturally low in fats and rich in vitamins, minerals, and phytonutrients promote arterial health and erectile success. These are the NO boosters. Next time you see your produce managers at the grocery store or farmer's market, give them the respect they deserve as unwitting sexual counselors.

ERECTILE DYSFUNCTION: A POWERFUL PREDICTOR OF SILENT HEART DISEASE

Erectile dysfunction is a powerful predictor of future coronary artery disease events. For example, if you live in Olmsted County, Minnesota, and are a man between the ages of forty and forty-nine without known heart disease but with ED, you have up to a fiftyfold higher incidence of eventually having new heart events compared to men the same age without ED. Rarely in medicine is there ever a risk factor this powerful. (By comparison, smoking may raise your risk of similar events threefold. Please do not smoke.)

WHAT TO DO IF YOU ALREADY HAVE ERECTILE DYSFUNCTION

Although this is a book on vegan sex, not vegan cardiology, my passion is to spread the love of both plant-based health and early heart disease detection. When ED is an issue, even when it precedes symptoms of heart problems, my advice is to see a physician, perhaps a cardiologist, interested in advanced detection and prevention of artery disease. This may not always be a way to get effective treatment, as sadly some doctors in primary care, cardiology, and urology are not aware of the established connection between the heart "bone" and boning. This is unfortunate, as there are extensive medical articles written on the topic that are available to all healthcare professionals. The most exhaustive medical reference is the *Princeton III Consensus Recommendations for the Management of Erectile Dysfunction and Cardiovascular Disease.*

In my preventive cardiology practice, I see patients who come solely for an evaluation of their ED, with no known heart issues. Most will have problems with blood pressure, blood sugar, or cholesterol; have a family history of heart disease or obesity; or all the above. The patients I see are going to receive information to address their diet, along with instructions for exercising regularly and practicing stress management, as I educate and guide them to an artery-healthy lifestyle that promotes a strong heart, rich production of NO, and a reliable erection. All the factors that matter for cardiovascular health will be measured. These can include blood pressure, weight, waist circumference, fasting blood sugar and insulin levels, total cholesterol and LDL particle number, hs-CRP for inflammation, homocysteine for methylation, and Lp(a) or lipoprotein (a), an inherited form of cholesterol that can clog arteries but is rarely measured. An EKG will also be performed.

As ED can be a clue to silent but serious heart artery blockages, I'll usually go a step further than just those tests. Generally I recommend that patients have a coronary artery calcium scan (CACS), which uses a modern high-speed CT scanner. It typically costs under $200 and is available at most local hospitals. You may have never heard of this test, but it's been around for over fifteen years and has thousands of medical research papers supporting it as the most accurate way to determine if the heart arteries are young, middle-aged, or old. It's a simple CT scan over the heart without an IV, iodine dye, or injection. There's a fascinating documentary called *The Widowmaker* that describes how this test was developed. Old heart arteries, even if silent in terms of symptoms, are calcified heart arteries, and they show up on the CT scan reliably. The whole test takes under a minute and results in a score that should be zero. If you want to score for a long time, you want a heart CT score of zero. It'll tell you that your ED is not due to advanced silent heart blockages, and that's great news. If the number is high—and it can be 200 or 2,000 even in active people, assuming they're otherwise healthy—then a protocol to halt and reverse heart disease with lifestyle and integrative measures can be implemented.

Only recently have we been able to approximate NO production by a simple blood test. Most doctors are not aware of it, and it's not available in all labs, but in my clinic I'll measure the level of a substance found in blood plasma called asymmetric dimethylarginine (ADMA). When this compound is high, it means NO production is low. When it's low, it means NO production is normal and high. It can also change quickly from abnormal to normal when a better diet, exercise, smoking cessation, and stress management are implemented along with some supplements, such as L-arginine. In addition, there's now a way to directly measure the health of the endothelium and its production of NO. This is called an EndoPAT (peripheral arterial tone) examination, and it requires an instrument that looks like a very fancy blood pressure cuff. I perform this noninvasive test in my office on men with ED to see if their endothelium is acting healthy or sick. I then prescribe a program for better arteries and better sex and recheck the patient in a few months.

To wrap up the connection between sex and the health of your heart, let's talk about a canary. In case you've never heard this piece of mining lore, a trick used by miners to avoid being exposed to and dying from elevated levels of toxic gases was to bring a caged canary into the coal mine. If the canary acted strange or died, the miners knew to exit the mine immediately before they were at risk for death, because the bird suffered the effects of the gases before the much larger workers. Erectile dysfunction is often referred to as a canary in the coal mine. The erection that doesn't happen or can't be sustained can give clues to a poor lifestyle and sick arteries three to four years before a heart attack strikes. Just like the miners fleeing the mine, you should run to a health-care professional familiar with the endothelium, NO, and ED and get a checkup. It might save your life and also restore your sexual performance and joy.

3 the physiology of sex and food

VEGANS, VAGINAS, VEGETABLES, AND VAS DEFERENS

by Joel Kahn, MD

Want hot, sweaty, passionate love up and down a staircase like in *The Thomas Crown Affair*? You can if your mind-set is right and your arteries and heart are acting youthful. Is vegan sex really the best sex in terms of the science of food and fornication? While there's been a lot of bravado and testimonials about the enhanced sexual prowess, longevity, taste, and general sexiness of those following a plant-based diet, does the science support it?

One of the most famous of the testimonials to vegan vigor in bed is found in the hit documentary *Forks Over Knives*. If you've never seen this classic, please watch it. Reference is made to the ability to "raise the flag" on a plant-based diet even in patients with advanced heart disease. People for the Ethical Treatment of Animals (PETA) has contributed to this banter with sexy ads submitted to the Super Bowl, but the ads were banned because they were just too steamy. They declared, "Go Vegan, Last Longer." Look for the short YouTube video on the web one night when the kids have gone to bed early. In the scientific arena, there's every reason to believe from a medical standpoint that vegan sex is the most reliable pathway to male and female potency and performance as we age.

Maybe you're wondering why you need to learn more about the physiology of sex and veganism if it's all working successfully for you. The sad truth is that there's such a high rate of problems with sexual performance that planning for the future is a smart idea even if you're a Tarzan or Jane right now. Indeed, your spoon can help you spoon far into the future.

There's more science to the sequence of events creating a male erection than there is for the female counterpart, so here's a brief and graphic rundown on how it all happens. If you're a visual learner and want a laugh-out-loud experience, check out Woody Allen's *Everything You Always Wanted to Know about Sex* (*But Were Afraid to Ask)* and look up the sperm scene. Here is the drier version:

1. Touch, sights, sounds, erotic memories, and fantasies cause sexual excitement.
2. These stimuli increase signal output from a part of the brain called the paraventricular nucleus. I love this part of the brain.
3. These signals then pass through special autonomic nerves in the spinal cord, the pelvic nerves, and the cavernous nerves that run along the prostate gland to reach the corpora cavernosa and the arteries that supply them with blood.
4. In response to these signals, the muscle fibers in the corpora cavernosa relax, allowing blood to fill the spaces within them if the endothelium is healthy.
5. Muscle fibers in the arteries that supply the penis also relax, and there's an eightfold increase in blood flow to the penis. The increased blood flow expands the sinusoidal spaces in the corpora, then stretches the surrounding sheath.
6. As the tunica stretches, it blocks off the veins that take blood away from the corpora cavernosa. This traps blood within the penis, the pressure becomes very high, and the penis becomes erect. This is ingenious. Let the red blood in and cut off the escape hatch for the blood in the veins.
7. During an erection, pressure in the penis is at least twice the pressure of blood in the main circulation. This is possible because the muscles of the pelvic floor contract around the base of the corpora cavernosa.
8. At orgasm, the signaling from the brain changes dramatically. There's a sudden increase in norepinephrine (adrenaline) production from nerves in the genitalia. This seems to trigger orgasm while also contracting the muscle fibers in the corpora cavernosa and their supplying arteries. As a result, the blood flow into the penis decreases.
9. The pressure within the corpora drops, which also relaxes the tunica, thereby letting blood flow out of the penis so it can again become flaccid. This is when some guys smoke a cigarette, but I advise against this Hollywood habit.

How big a problem is a penis that won't stay big? There are an estimated thirty million men in the United States alone with erectile dysfunction, and the problem is growing while the male organ is not. When sexual function falters, not only may romantic life suffer but overall health and specifically heart health can suffer too. As you now know, research shows that ED can be an early warning sign of heart disease. Words such as "sorry, I don't know what's wrong, but it's just not working like it used to" may forewarn of a heart attack three to four years in the future when no other problems in the present are apparent. Is it a coincidence that two medical terms of interest—endothelial dysfunction (poor artery health) and erectile dysfunction—are both abbreviated ED? In fact, if you want to be good in the B-E-D, you don't want either type of ED in your life. When there's ED (erectile dysfunction), there's ED (endothelial dysfunction) to blame. Healthy arteries are FUNdamental for a good, firm arousal and for swollen parts in both genders. Around three hundred years ago, Ben Franklin wrote that "an ounce of prevention is worth a pound of cure." Similarly, I tell my male patients, "To be older and hard, exercise daily and eat no lard!" Let's turn to some research on the relationship between dietary choices and successful sex, vegan style.

THE SEXIEST FOODS ARE PLANT BASED

Researchers from Harvard Medical School performed the first observational study of dietary habits and sexual function over a ten-year period just so you can pick foods for frolicking fun. The authors of the study estimated that over three hundred million men worldwide will soon suffer from erectile dysfunction and that vascular disease, or sick blood vessels, was a common cause linking ED to heart disease and stroke. They looked at 25,096 men from the Health Professionals Follow-Up Study, which was started by the Harvard School of Public Health in 1986. The study concentrated on how many servings these men were eating of plant-based foods, particularly those plant foods rich in flavonoid compounds known to be favorable to artery health. Although foods in grocery stores aren't labeled as being high in flavonoids, many of the foods you're probably already buying or growing are rich in these sexy compounds. These foods include apples, blueberries, citrus fruits (such as lemons and limes), and strawberries.

Every four years during the study, participants provided details of their diets and rated their erectile function (no pictures were required to be sent in). During the ten years of follow-up on these health professionals, a sobering 36 percent of the men reported erectile dysfunction. It appears that being a doctor isn't a guarantee of being immune to impotence. It also makes you wonder about taking advice regarding nutrition from many health professionals who have little education in the field and suffer the same consequences of the standard American diet as the rest of the population.

After additional factors known to be harmful to arteries supplying the sex organs (such as diabetes, high cholesterol, and smoking) were confirmed, dietary factors, including specific foods, were found to be associated with less ED, better erections, and better sex. The higher the intake of foods rich in certain flavonoid compounds (anthocyanins, flavanones, and flavones), the lower the risk of ED. If you remember only one lesson about eating for sexual health, make it this one: the higher the intake of fruit, the lower the risk of erectile dysfunction. To have a banana, eat a banana. Indeed, men eating the most fruit had a 14 percent reduction in their risk of ED over the ten years they were studied. It appears that if you add fruit today, you can keep the blue pill away. The Harvard data showed that eating apples, blueberries, citrus fruits, pears, and strawberries instead of chips, cookies, and fries can maintain normal sexual responsiveness. Therefore, I recommend that you make a firm commitment to eating more plant-based foods, particularly fruit.

Everyone can appreciate how sexy Europeans are, with their body-fitting clothes, positive perspectives on nude sunbathing, and acceptance of sex as a normal human function. It may be worth looking at some medical data from Europe, which we can use to maintain our own sexual prowess. Researchers at the Second University of Naples in Italy performed a series of studies on the Mediterranean (MED) diet and erectile dysfunction. The MED diet is a very plant-strong model to study, and there are versions that are "vegiterranean"—excluding meat and dairy and including only plant-based foods. In one study by Katherine Esposito, MD, the effect of a Mediterranean-style diet on ED in men was examined. All the men had a condition called metabolic syndrome, which involves a combination of abdominal obesity, high triglycerides, low HDL cholesterol, high blood pressure, and elevated blood sugar. Together, these factors predict increased cardiac risk. Sixty-five men with both ED and metabolic syndrome met the criteria. Half of them were assigned to eat a Mediterranean-style diet, and thirty were assigned to a control diet that included higher levels of meat and dairy, fewer whole grains, and less fruits and vegetables. After two years, men on the Mediterranean diet consumed more fruits, vegetables, nuts, whole grains, and olive oil compared to men on the control diet. Blood tests indicating healthy arteries improved in the MED diet group and were unchanged in the control group. There were thirteen men in the MED diet group and two in the control group who reported improved sexual function. Overall, the study suggested that a Mediterranean-style diet rich in whole grains, fruits, vegetables, legumes, walnuts, and olive oil might be effective in reducing the prevalence of ED in men with metabolic syndrome. I'm confident that adding these foods to the diets of anyone with ED, whether or not they have a diagnosis of metabolic syndrome, would enhance their ability to experience the joy of sex. The power of food to prevent and heal damaged endothelium and create more NO can result in better sexual responsiveness within just a few weeks.

How consistent is the data showing that the plant-based components of the MED diet may boost sexual performance? In a series of studies on 440 patients in Spain, there were 42 percent who reported ED. Factors related to ED, including diet and lifestyle, were studied. Patients with ED were more frequently sedentary people who smoked and consumed higher amounts of alcohol. Eating nuts and vegetables lowered the risk of ED by about half. Obesity, heart disease, and steady alcohol consumption were shown to be directly related to ED. Overall, erectile dysfunction was a very common disorder in these patients with risk factors for heart disease. Eating vegetables and nuts may be protective, as they are known to heal endothelium and drive NO production to higher levels.

The reason plant-based foods can quickly boost sexual function takes us back to endothelium and NO production, which is discussed on pages 12–13. The amino acids L-arginine and L-citrulline cycle back and forth and create NO in endothelial cells. This system is particularly active before the age of forty. A smart plan for maintaining peak sexual performance is to eat foods high in L-arginine that lead to NO production. If you occasionally eat almonds, Brazil nuts, peanuts, pine nuts, pistachios, and walnuts, you'll be getting L-arginine in your diet. If you're watching your weight (and who isn't!), be sure to limit nut consumption to about one small handful per day, as nuts are calorie dense. Whole grains, such as oats and wheat germ, also have significant amounts of L-arginine and should be a part of any healthy diet.

The amino acid L-citrulline, which is found in foods, can help arteries be responsive in order to support romance and passion.

Watermelon (particularly the white rind) has the highest concentration of citrulline in nature, and yellow watermelon is higher than red varieties. L-citrulline is also found in onions and garlic. Watermelon might be a better choice, however, before going on a date!

In addition to eating foods rich in L-arginine and L-citrulline to provide the building blocks for NO production, you can generate NO another way. There are chemicals called dietary nitrates found in many foods, such as beets and dark leafy greens, that can be converted in saliva to nitrites, absorbed, and then converted to NO. You can actually chew cruciferous vegetables and end up with the same reaction you might get from a prescription medication: more NO! Because this reaction requires the healthy mouth bacteria found in the grooves of our tongues, the process can be interrupted if you use antiseptic mouthwashes. These products can kill helpful bacteria and prevent healthy conversion of dietary nitrates to nitrites leading to NO production and successful sex.

The cruciferous vegetables that are rich in dietary nitrates include arugula, bok choy, kale, rhubarb, spinach, and Swiss chard. Beets can also supply dietary nitrates, whether they're eaten or juiced. "Beet off" takes on new meaning when you understand NO production! If you include apples, grapes, green tea, and pomegranates in your diet, you'll end up with a dynamite erotic potion.

Women also need blood flow for romance, and the same systems work in the female body, although they're studied less often in research protocols. There are limited studies using drugs like Viagra in women with diabetes and sexual dysfunction, and benefits were reported. As the mechanism used by Viagra to lead to sexual improvement has the same end result as NO pathways, it's reasonable to expect that women eating foods rich in L-arginine, L-citrulline, and dietary nitrates will experience a boost in their sexual responsiveness too.

Men often like to brag about their sexual prowess, whether that bragging takes place in the gym or the bedroom. This behavior frequently corresponds with eating steaks, smoking cigars, and watching football for hours while sitting on the couch—all activities likely to lead to less NO and more ED. In my opinion, the sexiest man is the one who loves animals but doesn't eat them and who takes care of his health by getting exercise and not smoking. This is true of women too. The best blue pill is a blueberry. The best aphrodisiac is a person who is kind to animals, takes care of the environment by making wise plant-based food choices, and enjoys the sexual benefits of plant-powered genitals.

A diet loaded with whole-food plants in place of animal-based foods may not reverse or prevent every single case of ED and female sexual dysfunction. If someone guarantees you 100 percent success, run the other way. Sex is simply too complicated. Even though sex is dependent on brisk and healthy blood flow redirection for male erection and female climax, it also has some components that even arugula and watermelon may not fix.

THE EFFECT OF A VEGAN DIET ON SEXUAL RESPONSE

We've learned a lot about the sexual response from the American research team of Masters and Johnson and their seminal (awkward word choice) work in the 1960s. They described the stages of the sexual response, and most of them, particularly the fifth one (a prolonged state of affection and desire), will smooth out with a smoothie. In fact, I think the best analogy to the Masters and Johnson formula is a smoothie. If you don't want to make one at all (Stage 5), why bother with the rest of the stages? But if you do, you need some interesting ingredients (Stage 1, arousal), some rather cumbersome planning reminiscent of cutting and prepping (Stage 2, plateau), activating the button (Stage 3, orgasm), and deceleration (Stage 4, resolution). Let's take our knowledge of making smoothies and blasts and apply it to the stages of your vegan sexual journey.

Stage 1: Arousal

This stage of sex is characterized by a rapid, sometimes super-rapid, response of the penis and female tissues to any and all excitement from visual stimuli (i.e., ogling), physical stimuli (such as holding hands, kissing, or grinding pelvic structures together on the dance floor), or psychological stimuli (such as loving emotions, which, I am told, may work if there's enough alcohol involved). As you know, arteries will dilate and blood flow will increase, permitting the swelling of sexual tissues with blood as manifested most obviously by an erect penis. This is one stage that a healthy lifestyle and diet will enhance.

During this stage, there's an increase in the heart rate and blood pressure, if the cardiovascular system is healthy and unencumbered by medications. Although this may sound like there's a lot of wiring and plumbing involved, this stage may happen in as little as thirty seconds, particularly if a Michael Bublé or Barry White song is playing. With age, medical conditions, or prescription drugs, the arousal stage may result in slower changes.

Stage 2: Plateau

Now that everything is swollen, wet, and primed for action, it would be a good time to remove some clothing or at least push some aside. With continued stimulation and no interference (cell phones, dogs, cats, children of any age, doorbells, work deadlines, to-do lists, unusual body odors, misplaced body hair, gas, itching . . . there can be a lot of distractions), the testicles will lift toward the body, the penis reaches full erection, and the number of breaths per minute peak to between thirty and forty. The healthier the heart and arteries, the easier this stage will be, so eat wisely.

Premature ejaculation in a man can interrupt this stage, so the key is to achieve control over it. A yoga practice concentrating on core strength is one type of exercise that can be practiced in order to prevent an early ejaculation. And as many yogis are vegan, we're back to your diet again.

Stage 3: Orgasm

This is a short stage, but I'm hopeful that genetic engineering or stem cell transplants may eventually extend this stage to hours or weeks (like the orgasmatron in the classic Woody Allen movie *Sleeper*). Orgasm happens with the rhythmic contractions of genital muscles that occur nearly every second and spread sensations throughout the entire body, including the overall sensation of the big O.

For men, orgasm includes ejaculation. Fatigue, alcohol, prescription medications, or someone knocking on the door can make it difficult for a man to finish ejaculating. It's possible that foods that diminish the health of arteries, even briefly, may prevent a successful erection and ejaculation. The Big Mac attack, for example, may indeed attack a man's ability to perform and leave him looking like Ronald the Clown.

The convulsions of muscles during orgasms, which are initially strong and then weaker (dammit), are said to be an expression of the quality of the orgasm. Others would argue that all orgasms are quality. During the peak of orgasm, usually lasting less than thirty seconds, heart rates may reach 160 to 180 beats per second and breathing rates may exceed forty per minute.

Stage 4: Resolution

What is the definition of eternity? A comedian would say that it's the time between orgasm and leaving your partner's apartment on a less-than-perfect date. Others might answer that it's the time it takes for a man to regain the ability to experience a successful erection and second orgasm. However, all good things must come to an end, and the intense blood flow to the genitals and the rest of the body following orgasm rapidly subsides. Peace has returned to the pelvic organs.

Stage 5: The First Stage, Sexual Desire

If you thought sex was confusing and at times frustrating, you're right. Indeed, the fifth stage of the physiology of sex actually occurs before the first stage and was added on after the publication of Masters and Johnson's research. Psychiatrist Helen Kaplan and psychoanalyst Harold Lief were the first to discuss the fact that 30 percent of patients seen in sexual consultancy complained of a lack of desire. There may be many reasons desire is absent, including mental and environmental issues. Desire is determined in part by attraction to the partner and deep-rooted fears, prior rejection, and feelings of guilt. The ideal state for successful and pleasing sex is a similar level of desire between the two partners (occurring every 1,012 years by astrological calculations). Sexual desire may also be affected by medications and medical conditions, such as heart disease and depression. Hormonal imbalances of the thyroid, adrenal glands, hypothalamus, and sexual organs may also be to blame.

One way to possibly enhance sexual desire is to ditch meat so you smell better. Yes, you read that right. There's science that indicates that non-meat eaters smell better and therefore are more attractive. Seriously? Seventeen male volunteers ate a diet of meat for two weeks and then a diet without meat for the same period. During the study, odor samples from the armpits of these men were collected and judged by thirty women as to the attractiveness of the smell. During the two weeks the men went without meat, the women judged the men's odors as more attractive, more pleasant, and less intense. You might meet the person of your dreams who raises your sexual interest if you stop eating meat.

Now that you understand far more about forks, knives, and fornication than you probably did before, let's talk about why sex may not only require a healthy heart but may also make your heart healthy.

THE HEALTH BENEFITS OF SEX

Heart health may result in great sex, but great sex can also lead to better health overall and longer life. Successful and vigorous sex is a part of many people's definition of health, and this is substantiated by science in so many ways. A study published in the *Harvard Health Letter* declared the following: "Sex is important to health. It revs up metabolism and may boost the immune system. Frequent sexual intercourse is associated with reduced heart attack risk." Sex also optimizes longevity. In a research project called the Massachusetts Male Aging Study, men who had sex once a month or less had a nearly 50 percent increased risk of developing heart disease compared with a group that had sex twice or more weekly. In another study, published in *BMJ*, over nine hundred men in Wales were followed for ten years; those with high orgasm frequency had 50 percent less risk of dying. If a participant had eight sexual episodes per month, the death rate was reduced by 36 percent, but the more often participants had sex, the lower the death rate dropped. Very few traditional medical therapies, such as medication or surgery, can boast lifesaving numbers like these.

Having sex on a regular basis can also lead to better brain function. In a study done in the UK, frequency of sexual activity corresponded with better cognitive function in older adults. Memory, executive function, and verbal fluency (all measures of brain health) were better among participants, both male and female, who had sex often. In another study done in Taiwan, sexual frequency in over two thousand men and women was inversely correlated with the blood concentration of an amino acid called homocysteine that may be bad for heart health. The more frequently participants engaged in sex, the lower their homocysteine levels were. There are other ways to lower homocysteine, such as taking B complex vitamins every day, but the data suggest you might just want to jump in the sack instead—and it would be a lot more fun.

Higher testosterone levels are associated with longevity, and a study done at Georgia State University shows that testosterone levels increase in men during intercourse with a partner. This occurs only with partner sex and does not necessarily rise during masturbation. Unfortunately, less medical data is available on the role of sexual frequency in female health, but there's a 2010 study that gives us reason to believe the advantages are much the same.

Finally, sex can reduce the risk of prostate cancer in men. A study analyzed by Harvard researchers assessed the frequency of ejaculation with prostate health and the development of prostate cancer. They discovered that the lowest rates of prostate cancer were found in men who ejaculated twenty-one times or more a month. That's only nine or ten days off a month, so these were very busy men.

The science is crystal clear. One of the best paths to a long and productive life is to view sex as a health-promoting activity. Schedule it on your calendar with the same priority you might mark down an appointment to work out with a trainer at the gym or take a yoga class. There's no doubt that when Marvin Gaye sang "Sexual Healing," he was teaching a medical truth.

4 good vegan love

by Ellen Jaffe Jones

Now that Dr. Joel has given a medical perspective on why being vegan leads to better sex and why better sex leads to better health, I want to share some insights both from me and other vegans on the relationships that nurture our sexual interactions. Sex with a vegan is great, but having a loving, intimate relationship with a vegan can make your entire life, not just your sex life, wonderfully fulfilling. If you want more altitude under the sheets, can you achieve that by elevating your purpose?

ATTITUDE IS ALTITUDE

I believe that partnerships, especially with vegans, can be exhilarating and beneficial to both parties in so many ways. When you find a partner who shares your values, it can be love at first and last sight—and everything in between. Having a vegan connection can take you to the mountaintop like nothing else ever will.

Veganism can be the cement that binds all the other components of a solid relationship. Vegan relationships that succeed do so largely because both partners are committed to serving the higher good, a cause, and being on the same side of the good fight. There are a number of vegan couples I know who glow like no others. The spark between them is like a thousand rays of hopeful light.

The ethic of veganism—which is more a lifestyle than just a diet—gives couples a feeling of freedom and power at the same time. Someone once described it to me this way: "Veganism transcends the physical. When both partners share the same values and ethics, it's a real turn-on. It keeps you in sync. Sharing higher values makes you feel more erotic and more sensitive to your partner's eroticism. Altruism becomes the motivating force in your lives. That can be very stimulating and never ending. It doesn't get dull."

Another pearl of wisdom was shared with me: "Serving the higher good is a real turn-on. You're focused outside of yourself and instead on other people and on saving animals. Your life becomes one of immersion in beauty, and that's a wonderful shared sensuality that never gets old. I want to implore people to go vegan and find a partner to share your vegan values with; then every day becomes much more exotic and erotic. You get to re-create every single day because you're sharing a common value. It's exciting."

If we're more tuned in to how animals think and feel, do we become more tuned in to our own animal-like behavior? Do we understand and connect to our behavior better because we see how animal-like it is? Perhaps. If we're more sensitive to nonverbal communication with animals, maybe we become more aware of how unspoken communication takes place between humans. When you care deeply about your partner's happiness, you sense their needs without having to ask. You instinctively and intuitively know when they need a hug or a peck on the neck.

Here's a testimonial from a man who went out with a vegan for the first time. It was their first date, and it was the first time he had ever met, let alone dated, anyone who was vegan. He noticed her eating a large salad and a lot of vegetables, then commented, "You're eating vegetarian, aren't you?" Men are so perceptive. She answered, "Why, yes. Actually it's vegan. Nothing with a mama or a face." She had liked her date up until then, and in somewhat stereotypical female apologetic fashion, she said, "But I don't shove it down anyone's throat." "That's good," he answered, not showing any inclination of wanting to know another thing about veganism. She figured, "OK, we're done." She didn't return his calls for a few weeks. When she did, all of a sudden he was interested in knowing more about her and her lifestyle. What a difference a little indifference can make. She took him under her wing, and the vegan tutorial took off. Six months later, here's the report from a smitten and changed carnivore:

> I spent the first seventy years of my life eating and enjoying meat, fish, and dairy like just about everyone I knew. I was taught by my parents, teachers, and church that *Homo sapiens* were meant to eat these things. I remember studying how our ancestors scavenged and hunted for their food. I learned how beef was raised and slaughtered

for the benefit of mankind. National health officials sent films about the "proper diet for healthy living" to schools. The famous food groups were displayed in triangles so they'd be easy to understand. When I was about twelve, my father took me to the infamous Chicago stockyards to see thousands of steer being led to their slaughter. Several of my friends were taught by their fathers to shoot a gun and go hunting, fishing, and trapping. I grew up firmly believing that this was the natural order of things. Man was on top of the food chain, and it was perfectly honorable to raise animals and fish for human consumption and mankind's survival. My mother even taught me how to select meat from the various cuts that were available in the markets.

I didn't question my elders, nor did I even think about it until I met a special person who took the time to enlighten me. It was very difficult for me to grasp the impact I was having on our environment. I also learned what damage I had been doing to my body over seventy years.

Now armed with this new insight, I was faced with the task of unlearning all that I had been taught and undoing all my habits and tastes. Slowly, very slowly, I entered into the vegan world. First, I stopped eating beef, fish, and poultry. Second, I stopped using dairy milk and butter, replacing them with similar-tasting vegan alternatives. Mayonnaise was the last to go. I won't kid you, it was tough to let go of what I thought was normal and tasted so good. I'm now a Vegenaise addict.

One thing from my prior diet was peanut butter. I didn't have to give that up; in fact, I ate even more of it. I learned about all kinds of plant foods that I had shied away from over the years and plants that I didn't even know existed. I not only learned about all the alternative foods that are now available, but I also learned about the health benefits associated with a plant-based diet.

As the months passed, I found myself still desiring my old standbys. I would order a hamburger or put a steak on the grill or sit down to a perfectly prepared swordfish or salmon dinner. Much to my surprise, those old familiar tastes were different. They weren't what I remembered. They were so much less than my expectations. The beef especially was almost revolting. Not only were my old favorite foods not pleasant, but they gave me gastric and abdominal pain.

After a few missteps, I began to notice the benefits of a plant-based diet. I'm not sure how to describe the conditions without stating them in graphic terms. My sinuses seemed to dry up. In the past, I would wake up in the morning and have to blow my nose two or three times in succession. I would spend the first half hour coughing up mucus that had accumulated in my throat during the night.

Having been a smoker for over fifty years, I was suffering from COPD and the beginnings of asthma. Once firmly on a vegan regimen, I realized better breathing capacity.

The best benefit I discovered was improvement of my sexual ability. I started to believe that, at seventy, my youthful sexual prowess was naturally fading. I was resigned to writing it off as old age. I found it more and more difficult to not only get an erection but also to sustain it. If I was lucky enough to have an erection and begin a sexual encounter, I would run out of breath and out of energy before the act concluded. It was very discouraging, to say the least. After about two months of eating a primarily vegan diet, I noticed that I was becoming more easily aroused to an erect state and that I could sustain the erection during a full and satisfying bout of lovemaking. I wasn't running out of breath, and I wasn't tiring due to the physical effort required.

I became more energetic. I wanted to do more activities. I began cycling on a daily basis. I kept increasing the distance of the bike rides, much to my surprise. I started feeling charged with energy. My attitude and outlook on life itself improved. I was no longer getting old. I was becoming incredibly revitalized.

On another note, my perspective on my environment changed too. I've always loved and cared for pets and enjoyed nature walks and birdwatching. I even volunteered at the local animal shelter. I just never associated love and compassion with animals that were intended for human consumption. I never even gave a thought to how the steer, lamb, pig, chicken, turkey, or fish got to my plate until I took the time to research it. What I found made me sad. I couldn't believe how the dairy, meat, and fish industries treat the animals and fish they produce for market. The way we can love our little puppy and allow such mistreatment of other animals is so incongruous.

In summary, my mind and my body have had a wonderful awakening. I intend to enjoy that body for many more years than I would have, given my former unhealthy way of life.

THE PROBLEMS WITH SITUATIONAL VEGANISM

It's been estimated that 70–80 percent of all vegans in the United States are women, and this percentage may grow as we get older. At many of the events I attend and observe, this statistic seems to hold. If you're dating women, there are likely to be a lot of options for you, but if you're dating men, finding the right vegan guy can be a challenge. How much can you encourage a significant other to adopt your vegan lifestyle and expect success?

Vegans Are Attractive

People who have it all in the vegan universe—they've become vegan on their own and are knowledgeable about and consistent with their vegan values—are irresistible. A partner you don't have to teach? That's beyond cool. No wonder they're sought after.

Some people get interested in veganism because their partner has brought them along kicking and screaming. If the relationship fails, often the partner who didn't come to the relationship as a vegan decides to go back to their former dietary habits. Sometimes they become vegan just to please their significant other. But as with so many things, you have to please yourself first. You can't get off any addiction—alcohol, tobacco, or animal products—because you want to please someone else. Having a partner you want to appeal to may be part of your motivation and inspiration to go vegan, but it can never be the sole reason. The decision to become and, more importantly, remain vegan for the long term must come from deep within. Successful commitment depends on how much your partner gets the message and is committed to the cause for all the right reasons, however he or she defines it.

I've seen an interesting thing happen to men who might be changing their diets for their women. Weeks or months after their conversion, they'll find themselves at a restaurant or public gathering digging into a pepperoni pizza or steak they really thought they were missing. The reactions on their faces when they experience stomach discomfort is memorable. They'll have an "aha" moment and say, "Ya know, I really don't like the taste of meat anymore." Hopefully they'll eventually get the vegan-for-animals connection, but as long as they hang on to a vegan diet, one more vegan in the world is always a good thing, no matter the reason.

People can and do change. It all depends on how much they want to be with you, which is often directly tied to their innate desire to please you. Sometimes their desire to go vegan is all about winning your favor. Go ahead and milk that one for all it's worth. But eventually, if the relationship lasts, they may take ownership of their journey to veganism and their justification for it. It's no longer so much about trying to please you as it is waking up one day and realizing, "Whoa, I feel better, I love better, and I love this food that I'm eating. And when I don't eat it, I feel like crap." All of a sudden, they understand how good it feels to regain their health and enjoy the community of others who share the same values and perspectives.

My hat's off to a guy I'd been seeing for a while who was real, honest, and direct. His daughter is a chef, and he raved about the plant-based meals she'd prepared for him. During a ten-day visit he and I had with his daughter, my friend joyously ate her food, commenting that he could eat vegan on a regular basis. Was it part of a courtship desire to impress me? Some of that was going on, I'm sure. But there was a real interest in exploring the terrain and enjoying improved health; if, in the process, it pleased me, so be it. I was game. Ultimately, as we all know, we have to be OK with our own choices.

As much as we may want to have a long-term relationship with another vegan, the heart wants what the heart wants, and we might find ourselves caring deeply for someone who doesn't share our life's passion for veganism. But the success of a relationship is measured more by whether both partners are equally committed to a life of service and are dedicated to using life's lessons to become better people—not so much whether they're committed to the same service. Perhaps your partner volunteers at the local homeless shelter, is active in politics, or leads a youth sports team. Even if their thing isn't particularly your thing, as long as you both respect each other's work and are supportive, your love can last and be inspiring to all around you.

VEGAN FOR HEALTH OR FOR ETHICS?

There's a study that shows that people who choose veganism for ethical reasons tend to stay vegan longer than people who change their diets only for health reasons. However, through my experience teaching cooking classes, I know many people who remained vegan for the long term because they had near-death experiences that motivated them to change their diets. As I'm fond of saying, people get desperate on their deathbeds. One woman, who'd been diagnosed with multiple myeloma (one of the more fatal forms of breast cancer) and was given little to no chance of survival, ended up in my PCRM Cancer Project cooking class. After eight months, she lost 120 pounds of extra weight, loved the food, and never counted calories. Thirteen years later, she's still alive and well, calling herself "a raving vegan."

I became friends with someone who was receptive to the vegan message because of his health problems. We began dating, and eventually he told me he hadn't had sex in a very long time—decades, in fact. Then he shared with me that he had a prescription for Viagra.

He tried using it a couple of times during our sexual encounters, but then, as you might expect, he no longer needed it. Not at all. And he never looked back. This, my friends, can be your story too.

VEGANS ON VEGAN SEX

I developed a survey to see whether men and women observed any physical or emotional differences in themselves after they became vegan. It's clear from so many respondents that being vegan makes a huge difference in their bodies, their relationships, and the sex they enjoy. The following are a few representative answers:

question: How long have you been vegan?

answer: Vegetarian with no eggs since 1987; vegan since 1993.

question: How long has your partner been vegan?

answer: Two years.

question: How was sex, specifically intercourse, for you before you became vegan? How was it for your partner?

answer: I wasn't having a lot of sex before I became vegan, so I'm not so qualified to comment. When I started having sex, I was already a vegetarian with no eggs and had been for a few years. I can say that being vegan gives me more confidence regarding sex because I've been told that I smell nice. I don't normally wear deodorant unless I know I'm going to be in an extremely stressful situation or am wearing polyester (which I tend not to wear). Lots of times when people hug me, they spontaneously say, "You smell good!" My husband also really likes the way I smell, and it's not because of a product. It's just that my diet has been pretty clean for a long time, so I don't smell the way I used to. When I was on the standard American diet, I most certainly needed deodorant!

question: Did you notice any changes in intercourse or sex in general after going vegan? If so, what were they?

answer: I was so close to vegan when I lost my virginity that I don't have any point of comparison.

question: Did you experience any emotional changes with sex after going vegan? If so, what?

answer: Again, I was almost vegan to begin with. The emotional changes I felt actually spread into every area of my life. When there wasn't any killing involved with what I ate, I felt so much better.

question: Do you believe that going vegan has created beneficial physical and emotional changes in your sexual relationships? If so, what?

answer: I don't know about sexual changes because of my lack of experience, but my endurance has gotten *so* much better since I became vegan. Sadly, I barely even move these days, much less exercise, but if I do end up going for a walk or bike ride, I can do it for a long time and not get tired. When I was veggie but not vegan, I trekked in Thailand. I was about twenty-six years old and was exercising a lot then. There were younger men (athletic—which I'm so not) on the trek, and I was always in the rear. Five years later, I was doing a more strenuous trek in Peru and hadn't exercised in a really long time, but I was vegan. There were athletic young men on that trek too, and to my great surprise, I'd be effortlessly in front of the pack.

question: Any advice for nonvegans about how sex might be enhanced if they went vegan?

answer: Life, in all aspects, is enhanced by being vegan. There's a deep joy in being kind to animals and the planet. Also, being vegan really does make people smell better and feel better. I can't imagine having sex after eating animal products—probably feeling bloated, enervated, gassy . . . so not romantic. Feeling underlying guilt about doing heinous things to fellow beings. I have literally cried many tears about eating so many animals growing up—so much blood on my hands before my wires connected regarding this issue. I'm so glad my kids are lifelong vegans so they don't have to carry this subconscious load.

another response: I was first married to a man seventeen years younger than me. Since my current husband is five years older than I am, there was a difference of twenty-two years in terms of age and maturity between the two men. I don't want to embarrass my spouse (now a vegan), but he has a lot more vigor than my first husband! The first spouse was an omnivore and was beginning to lose his sexual vigor in his early forties. He ate a lot of fish and cheese. My current husband is now in his mid-fifties with no signs of slowing down in that area. It's an unexpected blessing to be with a vegan male, and I try to make this point with others as a "selling feature," without being too graphic. All about the blood flow? That's right! My husband is very shy and would never discuss his activities with others, but I feel this is an important point to make. ED is a sign of a faltering vascular system, as you know, of course. It's not just a normal part of aging.

My survey showed me that both vegan men and women feel sex is inspired on a deeper level than titillation. While provocative images and memories are key to stimulating basic animal arousal, what makes humans different from other animals is that we have the ability to process, think, and feel in ways that are unique to our species. We can override our most selfish instincts to experience pleasure and show concern for others. We can also opt to be completely selfish and choose how we live our lives based on our subconscious needs.

If we're working toward a higher good—and our priority is trying to eliminate suffering on all levels—then what we wake up and do in the morning becomes a fairly easy decision. Who we hang out with becomes easier. Who we have sex with becomes a no-brainer. Dedication to a cause does become the glue that holds our partnerships together.

INSIDE THE MALE AND FEMALE BRAIN

You want a good vegan relationship and perhaps the sex that comes with it. But have you felt clueless about how to maintain a relationship? Is the male or female mind a complete mystery to you? Do you think men and women are, or should be, alike?

I pretty much get me—and my mother, sisters, daughters, and all the women friends in my life. But men? That's another story. In the course of my journey, and in part because I was starting to write this book, I began researching the male brain and behavior in earnest. I did learn a few things and discovered patterns of male behavior—and in the process discovered some patterns in women too.

Men do think often about women and sex, like every seven seconds or seven minutes, whichever statistic you want to believe. The thought process is tied more to their anatomy and not their brains. Sometimes it's described bluntly: men think with their penises. They're hardwired to be attracted to women in a big way.

The game of courtship brings out a certain amount of creativity and romanticism in both sexes. Men usually resort to physical activity to please their partners. He'll build. He'll buy flowers. He'll rearrange or buy furniture to feather the nest. He'll tear out the landscaping and weed like there's no tomorrow. He'll text photos of all his efforts to prove his undying love, in case you're not there to witness them.

Then there are moments The Penis takes over. He'll respond to graphic images of scantily clad nude women that appeal to his basic instincts. Or as Dale Alderman in his book *Everyday Dad* described it, "a man's brain has two lobes: the 'Oh yeah, baby, I'm thinking about sex lobe,' which takes up 88 percent of the brain, and the 'Future Sites of Dreams' about supermodels, which takes up 10 percent. The 'Everything Else' takes up 2 percent. The broadband connection in women's brains allows them to multitask. In a man's brain . . . we can only focus on one task at a time, and if we are interrupted while we are working on the task, our brain experiences a fatal error." I'm so glad that was written by a guy taking ownership.

Growing up during the sexual revolution, I was taught to believe in the equality of the sexes and that there aren't significant differences between men and women—or that there shouldn't be. However, I have three daughters and my sister-in-law has four sons, and they're all about the same age. I resisted believing there was any difference between the sexes until I saw it play out among these kids. When her kids came over, the boys would beat up on each other and tear apart toys and furniture. As best they could, my girls tried to play quietly with their dolls and books and engage in more sedate activities. But sometimes even my girls got drawn into the brawls; one of them ended up with stitches from a fall off of a chair. My sister-in-law and I joked that each visit ended up with a few hundred dollars' worth of damages.

Into adulthood and through multiple relationships, I've observed that guys love to be physical, be it sports or anything that involves motion. When the going gets tough, generally, they hate talking about it. The less time spent talking about relationships or emotions, the better. If there's a problem, they prefer to either run or engage in sports or go out to the garage and fix a piece of furniture or equipment or a vehicle. Give them a few days or weeks to fix or landscape a house, and bliss sets in. Help them with those projects in some small or big way, and they'll like, love, or at least remember you forever.

Go to a man with a problem, and he'll want to fix it; go to a woman with a problem, and she's happy just to hear you out and commiserate with you. Men are practical; they want things to work. Women need beauty in their surroundings. Things that are pleasing to the senses don't have to have a practical purpose. If men are thinking about the future, they're making plans; women like to dream about what might be possible.

There are *always* exceptions to this pattern, and this can be as confounding to men as to women. Think of the big, strong guy who's

Romance in the Kitchen

To a vegan man, having a hot meal prepared a couple of times a day—or even a week—is nirvana. While this is really old school, it's true that the way to a man's heart is through his stomach. Spoiler alert: This works for women too. There's nothing more appealing to a vegan woman than a thoughtful, compassionate man who can prepare a delicious vegan dinner all on his own.

For busy men or women, any kind of help is welcome. If you enjoy cooking, by all means share your love and enthusiasm in the kitchen. Don't hesitate to build your partner's confidence, however. If he or she lacks experience cooking, assign simple tasks, such as mincing onions or garlic, to build confidence and foster a partnership based on cooperation and lifelong learning.

very attuned to relationships and finds it important to talk about how the people around him are getting along. Then there's the take-charge gal who's as eager to compete and make stuff as any guy is and thinks that trying to understand a complex, emotional mind is a total chore. There are definitely guys who are dreamers and women who are doers.

Just know that there *are* tendencies, so be aware of them. So much of what people fight about in a relationship has root causes in the differences between the sexes. No, he's not an insensitive jerk; worrying about how your kids are getting along with their best friends is simply not something that's high on his list of priorities. You're not annoying by insisting that he put on a clean shirt and pants when he goes out with you; you just want him to look attractive and, by association, make you look and feel better when you're with him. I think every high school should add a "men and women are from two planets" class to its curriculum so more people could start their social lives with a better understanding of what makes the other sex tick. All for world peace!

VEGAN AS YOU AGE

Both women and men can experience a vegan advantage as they approach their golden years. Better health increases the chance that both partners will be able to enjoy activities together for years to come, including an active sex life. But the realities of aging often do set limits. How can those limits be managed?

For women, menopause doesn't have to mean an end to sexuality. In fact, not having to worry about birth control is often a freeing feeling and allows you to be more spontaneous with your partner without worrying about reproductive consequences. However, the change in hormones after menopause can affect even vegan women, although some studies show that a plant-based diet can reduce the onset of hot flashes and vaginal dryness and maintain the thickness of vaginal tissue. However, if diet and lifestyle changes are not enough, you should know that a lot of progress has been made in the area of hormonal supplementation.

After some scares about increased risk of heart attacks with hormone use, more positive outcomes were seen with plant-based bioidentical estrogen, progesterone, and testosterone. This is particularly true when estrogen is applied transdermally, as a cream, rather than taken orally, because when estrogen circulates in the bloodstream, it's processed by the body without dangerous effects to the heart. That's not the case when it's ingested and makes its way to the liver. If you find your libido is low, night sweats are waking you up at all hours, and intercourse is painful, look for a health professional in your area who's knowledgeable about testing hormone levels and supplementing with hormones to get you back to safe levels. If you've had cancer, especially breast cancer, be sure your provider takes this into account and will prescribe for your individual situation.

This same advice holds true for guys. Maybe you're not as interested in sex as you used to be, you're having a harder time getting hard—or maybe you're having more trouble kicking colds and healing from aches and pains than you used to. Testosterone aids in the regeneration of muscles and tissue in addition to providing a boost to libido and occasionally helping to improve erectile function. If you have elevated PSA levels, discuss with your health provider whether testosterone supplementation is appropriate for you. Researchers used to be concerned that increased testosterone would cause prostate cancer, but now it's believed that this is only a problem if a man already has prostate cancer.

What if you have a stellar diet but you still experience ED? It does happen, and it can be discouraging to feel as though there's no reward for all your diligence. My advice? Take matters into your own hands and experiment with all the different ways you can be physically affectionate with your partner. Don't be shy about communicating your needs. Maybe it'll be easier for your partner to reach orgasm than it is for you, and although you love them deeply and want to make them happy, let them know how they can satisfy you in turn. Even if intercourse is no longer possible, be sure to have some naked time together. Forget the pj's occasionally, or take a bath or shower together every once in a while. Break out the massage oil and rub out the stresses of the day. Kiss each other all over. Guys might think there's no point in physical intimacy if there's no ejaculation at the end of it, but even the biggest and toughest males need to be nibbled on now and then.

PLAN ON GROWING OLD

While many vegans have nonvegan partners, it's important for them to look down the road and consider the statistics on life expectancy. There certainly are meat eaters who are vigorous into their nineties, but they're the lucky few. Having a diet high in animal foods increases the risk of health disasters that can wreak havoc on a relationship—physically, emotionally, and especially financially. As we get older, we hope to have a partner who will still be with us. Injury and loss occur more frequently with age, and going through the resulting trauma can help us realize how life can be taken away at any moment.

On a subconscious level, even the strongest and most independent of us has an innate need to be nurtured and cared for, and that feeling of need seems to increase with the years. You may find yourself caring for an aging partner who's suffering from chronic illness at a time when you had hoped they would be around to enjoy an active lifestyle with you and support you. Not having someone to look out for you while you care for someone else takes an immense toll, especially if your partner is ill for a number of years. Having a vegan partner can be somewhat of a life insurance policy. It won't prevent the inevitable, but it may help to delay it.

IS VEGAN FOR LIFE SOMETHING YOU SHOULD EXPECT?

Many animal species partner up for life for mutual protection, food gathering, and child-rearing. The term "empty nester" evolved because even after child-rearing is done and the nest has emptied, animal parents may still stay together.

Our changing expectations about lifelong partnerships have a lot to do with the evolving role of women and their growing indepen-

PETA's Pitch for Vegan Sex

Because this chapter is all about the positive, let me share some humor with you. As we've mentioned, People for the Ethical Treatment of Animals (PETA) is known for its effective and memorable public service ads and increasingly in-your-face commercials. One of its most controversial commercials was banned from the 2016 Super Bowl, but you can still watch it on YouTube. Look for it under the title "Last Longer PETA commercial."

The ad shows a split screen with two couples presumably having intercourse between strategically placed sheets. The guy, who's a meat eater, can't sustain an erection or climax. He dies a mortifyingly quick sexual death, and his female partner storms off in frustration. Meanwhile, the vegan couple is still going at it, moaning away until the end of the commercial when a banner plasters the screen saying, "Last Longer. Go Vegan."

PETA has been trying long and hard, literally, to get a commercial like this on the Super Bowl because of the game's large TV audience. But getting an industry like advertising, which is bought off by the meat and dairy industries, to relinquish its choke hold on the truth and run the ad was and still is a problem. But no matter. These rejected ads get almost as many viewers eventually on YouTube and other social media platforms.

If you search for "vegetarians have better sex" on YouTube, you'll come up with another rejected Super Bowl ad showing scantily clad women losing strategically placed clothing and having erotic interactions with produce, such as pumpkins and asparagus. But don't stop there. Be sure not to miss the one called "Penis Inspired New 2012 Provocative Advert" produced by PETA UK. This is a classic, played out by old and young men alike. They're all fully clothed, but with carrots, cucumbers, eggplants, and bananas nestled in "hairy" collections of lettuces and escarole—and somehow attached to their crotches. Once in a while a flash of a couple of limes and oranges, standing in for testicles, poke out, as these wildly energetic men dance at car washes, on tennis courts, and along sidewalks. It's hard to watch this just once! The message "Increase Your Sexual Stamina" is followed by the finale, "Go Vegan."

dence. The vow "until death do us part" was once vital because it instilled an expectation that a man would provide for his female partner beyond child-rearing. Life expectancy in the early 1900s was in the mid-forties; currently that's almost doubled. At the same time, women have become more self-reliant and gained the skills to support themselves. Is it realistic to think that people can maintain a relationship spanning six decades or longer?

Sometimes my research brings me to the conclusion that men are biologically programmed for multiple relationships. It can be difficult for some of them to settle down with one person for the rest of their lives. Not to say it doesn't happen. Take my folks, for example. They were together for sixty-four years. It wasn't until elementary school that I realized they had different first names. It was a sad day for me when I was told they weren't both named "Honey," as I had put down on a school form. Having that kind of love and devotion as a role model can be as challenging as it is inspiring.

But again, stereotypes aren't always accurate. For every guy who gets the itch and wants a change of pace, there's another guy who likes things just the way they are, thank you very much. There's wisdom in this old adage: "Women marry men hoping to change them. Men marry women hoping nothing will change." Switching that up, there are also women who tire of the same social scenery day in and day out and are hoping for something better—or at least something different. Some people hold hard and fast to the romantic notion that love should be eternal, and for them the journey is as enjoyable as the launch.

Maybe you can think of people as being either trees or birds. Tree people love putting down roots. They derive pleasure from observing the change of seasons from the same spot, while growing both higher and deeper—and reaping the benefits of both altitude of viewpoint and depth of stability. In their relationships, tree people marvel at how both they and their partners change with the years, and they enjoy finding new ways to love each other as they evolve. Bird people fiercely protect their freedom to go where they need and want to. If they have to keep on the move, that's fine with them. Life isn't about one place or one person; it's all about the journey and delighting in all the possibilities that could be enjoyed. They relish a satisfying relationship, but there's always an expiration date.

No judgment here. We're all different and have different needs. Rather, I hope the insights I've gotten from my vegan relationships and vegan friends can help you get the most out of the good love you share.

5 when good vegan love goes bad

by Ellen Jaffe Jones

Just because you're vegan, doesn't mean you'll always have stellar sex, and just because you've picked a vegan partner doesn't guarantee a long and happy relationship. Your romantic dream of a blissful pairing might be a Disney fantasy, but how it actually plays out is a reality TV show—including all the drama that comes with it. No matter how we justify it, breakups are painful and not how we thought the script was written. What gets in the way of good vegan sex and why can it go wrong?

DEALING WITH THE COMEDOWN

In each of my marriages and in some of the relationships I had before and after them, erectile dysfunction was part of the equation. It was almost as if it was part of the aging process (even though onset at age twenty-eight seemed a bit young!). I accepted ED as a way of life. Gone were the virile men of my twenties and thirties. By forty, my partners were truly over the hill. The idea of geriatric sex became an oxymoron; who in an aging population addicted to meat and dairy could get it up enough to get it on?

As the abilities, and then interest, of my sexual partners declined, we both started making excuses and creating rationalizations for the problem. "Not tonight, dear. I have a headache" turned into "It's OK. Whatever you do or don't do is fine with me. No judgment here." And finally, "You know, what matters is emotional intimacy, friendship, and compatibility. Sex is greatly overrated anyway."

My partners were heavy meat and dairy eaters before I went vegan, for sure. After I went vegan, they would say that they ate a healthy diet, but in all cases, they still consumed some fish and dairy. Before I knew about the connection between heart health and ED—and how diet drives both—I, like so many other women, kept agonizing about the underlying cause of my partners' inabilities to perform. Sometimes women believe there's something wrong with them when their man isn't happy, and they'll run to a therapist to fix what they think is broken from within.

Was it possible that my partners and I weren't happy with each other and that's what instigated the problem? Or was their failure to perform not caused by their feelings but mostly, or totally, by the condition of their bodies? I wondered if my partners transferred their own feelings of inadequacy to criticism of me? How much did an animal-heavy diet block their arteries, including those in the brain? Did erectile dysfunction make them suspicious, constantly accusatory for no valid reason, and eventually nasty and violent? Was ED truly at the root of our worst problems?

One former partner with ED told me I was too emotional and needed to think more rationally, like him. Did he just not get that this is often how the two sexes split the division of emotional labor? Or, in my passion to give as much as I could to the world, or with my enthusiasm to live life to the fullest, did I expect too much and forget to take my theoretical chill pill?

Our physical quirks often drive our emotions in ways we're only just beginning to understand. As PCRM's Neal Barnard, MD, often points out, the excessive amount of testosterone that circulates in the body from an animal-heavy diet contributes to anger issues in some men. It could very well be that this, combined with feelings of inadequacy from ED, drove my partners to be critical of me and their situation in life.

BEING VEGAN DOESN'T ENSURE A HEALTHY OUTLOOK

There's nothing like the high you can get from falling in love with a vegan. I once was in a restaurant with a vegan love when our server noticed the vegan message on my companion's shirt. The server began peppering him with questions about what it was like to be vegan. Without missing a beat, he answered a dozen questions citing research, experience, and how much he enjoyed making a

Is Monogamy a Myth?

Why is it that people can be so confused about what they want in a relationship? In one conversation, they may tell you that they're looking for a soul mate, and you're as darned close as anybody has come in the last half century. But when someone else desirable appears, you discover you're not really the one and only.

What makes one person monogamous and another not? It's often hard to say. Relationship-aversion behavior can be indicative of someone who can't commit for all kinds of reasons, none of which have anything to do with veganism. My short answer is that when someone has a rugged breakup and is deeply hurt, they're more open to doing what it takes to please a person in the next relationship. However, if they've always been the one doing the breaking up, even if they're a compassionate vegan, they may not understand how awful being dumped can be or may not be invested enough in relationships to make a go of them.

connection to people about vegan benefits. I remember an almost out-of-body experience watching us all at the table. I felt so proud and happy and grateful that I could relish and take in the moment. I've never felt so in sync with anyone.

When the relationship crashed and burned, I couldn't understand why. What did I miss? How could he let it go? Didn't he know how good he had it? I egotistically asked myself (and asked him once too), "How could anyone else be as good as me?"

Consider yourself warned that having a vegan partner is no guarantee against heartbreak. If anything, it can be as tough as any relationship you'll ever experience—maybe more so—because you thought your mutual veganism (your shared beliefs, values, and common goals) made a bond stronger than superglue.

Vegans tend to be especially caring and compassionate, and I've seen more than one fall victim to someone who was trying to avoid dealing with early childhood hurts or adult traumas. Emotional injuries that happen in early childhood—the loss of a parent, for example—can have a big effect on relationships later in life, and the affected person may end up playing the role of an abandoned child. Veganism can also be used to cover or camouflage a deep hurt that's never been properly addressed. While some people are great at compartmentalizing and putting trauma in a shoebox on a high shelf, others are the walking wounded, wearing heartaches and neediness on their sleeves.

While I believe the tendency to prey on victims who've chosen the cause of veganism as an escape isn't common, it's definitely something to be aware of, especially if you feel you may be vulnerable. Individuals who prey on the weak can use veganism as a cover to gain favor. They'll pick someone who's chosen veganism as a way to alleviate the pain and suffering experienced in an earlier traumatic event—which might have even been witnessing abuse to animals or humans or both. The images, sounds, and feelings generated by that event may recede into the background, but they never completely disappear, making these people susceptible to someone who promises them special attention. I recall a story about the president of a vegetarian club who was ousted from his position when it became obvious he was using his power to make sexually inappropriate advances toward female club members. This can happen in any organization.

Even vegans have inner demons they must wrestle with and fix themselves. No one else can mend the effects of a painful childhood or a bad or even mediocre marriage.You can only give it your best shot. Knowing when to leave is part of the self-respect you owe yourself.

To the extent someone is truly looking for a partner, only you can decide how much energy and time you want to devote to making that possibility a reality. We're all invested in our egos and beliefs about ourselves. If we believe positively in ourselves, as we're always told to do for healthy self-esteem, we can end up wondering why some relationships don't work out. Your partner may tell you it's not you, it's them, and that might be true. You may have been the best catch in the world, but your partner wasn't ready for you and maybe never will be, no matter what they say. Maybe you just weren't a good fit, or maybe you weren't too anything at all. Maybe it really was never about you to begin with.

HOW TO BE OVER IT WHEN IT'S OVER

So, for whatever reason, that great vegan relationship is over. You may argue with yourself and wonder if you'll ever be able to move on or whether you will be stuck in this emotional crevasse forever. You can stomp out a flame, but the coals and embers are more challenging. They ignite just when you think the last one is gone. We'd all be in worse shape than we are if the truism "time heals all" wasn't actually true. The brain is an amazing manipulator of emotion, and with enough time and self-talk, you may be able to wiggle out of that seemingly endless canyon of heartache.

Millennials Give Sex a Cold Shoulder

Recent studies show that millennials (people born between 1980 and 2004) aren't all that interested in sex, especially not as much as generations before them. Pundits give all kinds of possible reasons, such as they have nothing to prove or they just prefer to work on a career instead of a relationship.

There are many studies, reports, and articles showing that the more we're connected online, the less we're connected in real life. How often does it happen that people sitting right next to one another text to communicate? Texting instead of talking gives people a way to hide from each other while also letting them have total control of their messages. An old-fashioned phone call or face-to-face chat might be more scary and revealing, given that there are audible and visual cues that can direct the conversation. This means that members of a younger generation are losing their ability to look into their partners' eyes and talk directly to them. They've isolated themselves, even from the ones they love. Being "out of touch" has grown in meaning.

Pregnancy—a potential outcome of having sex—might not be appealing to millennials if they're concerned about what kind a world will be around in twenty, forty, or sixty years. If the future of the planet involves environmental degradation and seemingly unstoppable conflict, many young people are asking, "Who would want to bring children into such a world?" Social media can be a great educational tool, but it also amplifies the stark reality of the future that lies ahead for the planet.

The technology of social media allows anyone to check up on an ex and see if they've found someone new. Sadly, you could drive yourself crazy by thinking, "They like that dingbat better than me?" Don't. Just don't. Move on. Be done. I realize that's *so* much easier said than done, but there are other vegans at the sanctuary, so to speak. Hone those compartmentalizing skills. Put the relationship to one side and don't ever look at it again. I remember hearing that 50 percent of popular songs are about relationship breakups—so pick a few. Roll up your car windows and sing and cry loudly. Let the healing begin. There's value in that pity party. Many of us have been there, and it's hard to pick up the pieces and move on. Better that than to wallow in toxic relationships.

I still mourn over the loss of certain guys I cared about, but I do that less and less as time goes on. Perhaps because I loved as a vegan and have loved other vegans, the glue that held us together was that much harder to crack. However, it's the vegan connection that may keep us together as friends. No matter what else happens, I've always felt glad about that. The further I get from the heat of the moment, the more I recognize that those relationships were flawed. The guys I dated spent a lot of time caring about themselves and showed an acute lack of interest in my life, rarely asking me how my life was going or being there for me when things got tough. Being vegan led me to be so optimistic that it clouded my judgment. Lesson learned: be ever vigilant.

Friends will tell you you're way too cool and awesome to remain stuck on anyone who doesn't appreciate or love you for who you are. But accepting that is much easier said than done, isn't it? Maybe you tell yourself it was just a transitional relationship. Maybe it freed you from an unloving partner, perhaps a carnivore who had no respect for your developing beliefs, and that lost relationship moved you further along to something better. Sounds a lot like the sales training I got on Wall Street—it takes forty nos to get one yes. A phone slammed down in your ear is all that much closer to the next yes. Again, would that it would be so easy.

Having a strong, viable partnership can be important to people who want to help animals, improve human health, and save the environment. But after a few of my own harsh experiences, I can understand why some people find themselves so involved in animal rights—they just give up on caring for people. It's so much easier to love a peaceful animal than a human being who talks back, argues, abuses, disrespects, or doesn't appreciate. Animals love unconditionally. What's not to love about that? It's also way easier (and better for you) to focus on a cause higher than yourself than to stay too long at that pity party.

While some of what I've shared has explored the negative experiences of having a vegan partner, the potential pitfalls involved are well worth the incredible highs of being with someone who's in sync with your values, goals, and dreams. There's nothing like it, and you'll know when you're there. You may have to kiss a few frogs to find your prince or princess, but hang in there for a while and know that if you want that vegan partner, it can happen. It's *so* worth it!

6 stories of love and loss

by Ellen Jaffe Jones

I've been married several times and have had numerous relationships, as many people do by the time they mature. Through the years, I've shared my stories of love and loss with my family, friends, and fellow vegans and have gotten a variety of reactions to them. One of my children told me, "Well, Mom, at least that means you've been loved that many times. Some people never know love." Great. I guess. OK. I'll take that to the bank.

But most of the people who've heard these tales have been fascinated and stunned and can totally relate to the changes I went through. Many have urged me to write a book about these romantic misadventures, and to that end, here they are. These four stories are raw, honest, personal, and candid. They speak to men and women, particularly vegans, who've been deeply hurt in a relationship and aren't sure why. Maybe if we talk more about how we've been treated, we can learn something from it and treat others with more emotional intelligence as a result.

Spoiler alert: Being vegan doesn't make you a whole person. It doesn't protect against the atrocities and damage that may have occurred earlier in life and that make it hard for someone to build a long-term relationship. Just because your partner is vegan doesn't mean you're guaranteed a life of bliss, ideal companionship, and wild and crazy love in and out of bed. Vegan relationships are as varied as the food on our plates. Long-term success is still determined by the factors that hold any successful relationship together: trust, respect, deep commitment to pleasing and honoring the other, a sense of fun, and putting the needs of the other person before oneself. Veganism is but one large piece of a huge puzzle.

You would think that the very definition of veganism would automatically make a vegan more loving, compassionate, giving, feeling, and caring. If someone cares enough about helping animals, then it would seem logical that they would treat humans with equal compassion. Sometimes yes. Sometimes no. Humans are complex. A person with unhealed emotional wounds may consciously or unconsciously use animals to heal from failed relationships. Animal causes may give them a safe haven and a respite from a cruel and unkind world. They may prefer the protection and unconditional love animals provide over the risky behavior we humans offer. The animals don't mind where our heads are at as long as we care. They have little interest in whether we figure ourselves out. Some days I wake up and think that it might be easier to start a relationship with someone who isn't vegan but is open to information and that I could just connect the dots for them. The gratitude someone feels when they've improved their health as the result of your example is one of the most rewarding feelings you could ever experience. There is no finer paycheck.

Before I launch into my stories, let me explain why I characterize my former partners the way I do. I don't want to identify the individuals involved; I just want to give my own version of what happened. The names have been changed to protect the not so innocent. And to further blur the lines between men I've been married to and my significant and not-so-significant others, I'm using the word "ex" to apply to all of them. That's your roadmap; let me take you on my journey.

SUSTAINING A MEAT EATER

It's important to know what you're getting yourself into if you choose a partner who isn't vegan, shows no interest in becoming one, and has one or more of the diseases of dietary overabundance, such as cancer, diabetes, and heart disease. The relationship with one of my exes eventually ended for the most part because he didn't respect my veganism and probably many other things about me as well.

He and I discussed my growing vegan passion, which was initially fueled by my own health concerns. He chuckled, recalling that when he went to various doctors to get treated for heart disease, they told him his failing penis may have been the first clue that his heart was in poor shape. Even after these warnings, he remained in denial. He'd tell friends that he didn't have heart disease, even though he'd been on blood thinners, blood pressure meds, and cholesterol-lowering drugs since we first met decades earlier. When I tried to give him some advice about how to adopt a plant-based, heart-healthy diet, he couldn't go there. When I would confront him about his denial, he would simply say, "I haven't had a heart attack, so I don't have heart disease."

I promote veganism wherever I go and often strike up conversations with the curious. He grew weary of the same questions that came my way and my same answers. As my health and athleticism continued to improve, his declined. Then the inevitable happened: he had a major heart attack. His fat-clogged arteries were screaming for bypasses. After he was treated and released, his resentment seethed below the surface at first and then became blatantly obvious, especially when a friend asked him point blank why he just didn't eat what I made. In short, my thriving on a vegan lifestyle was a threat and a constant reminder to him of how his own lifelong choices had failed him.

Like many other women, I was committed to doing whatever I could to help him eat healthy food. I was always happy to fix him mostly vegan meals and even willing to prepare fish when he refused to eat vegan main dishes (which was most of the time). In our divided dietary household, I would fix him vegan side dishes, which tended to be mostly grits and occasionally a whole grain. After he had his heart attack, one of the doctors asked when he last ate something green, as in a vegetable. He laughed and said he couldn't remember. But at least I had tried with all my heart, using the best information I had.

I knew something else was seriously wrong with our relationship. The constant fighting, the cantankerousness, the edginess, the combativeness—I believe all of these were a direct result of him not getting much satisfaction physically and emotionally. When confronted, he would blame his bad treatment of me on his mother and ex-wife. In joint therapy, he would be reminded that I was neither of those two women from his past and was actually a pretty nice, thoughtful gal who was a part of his current life.

The increasing hostility my ex developed over my veganism became painfully and embarrassingly evident and visible in public. He grew increasingly intolerant and impatient when I included animal rights in my vegan-for-health talks. Even though his friends and health-care professionals told him that to avoid continued heart disease and another heart attack, he ought to go easy on or give up the consumption of animal foods in favor of plants, at some point, it no longer mattered to him.

But even before the heart attack, his support of my activities waned. Not once did he ever suggest going to a vegan restaurant, and when I made the suggestion, he nixed it. I should have left in those moments. But because of our committed relationship, which was not easy to toss aside, I kept hoping. And hoping. Like so many women, I thought I could fix it if I made the right meal, did the right thing, and kept on smiling.

Eventually, the thought of relinquishing my relationship to my growing vegan passion certainly crossed my mind. Did my "cult" claim our relationship, as my ex would accuse? Did I lose my partner to veganism? I wondered in my darker moments. Truth was, the real reason I left was because the effects of his disease made him delusional and eventually violent. After going through hell and back, I decided that veganism was not to blame and vowed I'd never again live with anyone who wasn't vegan.

LOSING MY VEGAN VIRGINITY

You would think that the vegan connection, once cemented, would be forever. Until death do us part, or somewhere along that continuum. Warning: The pain of breaking up with someone who is vegan, combined with all the other stuff that melds a solid relationship, is also like no other.

Getting It Up to Get It On

This may be the most personal and intimate part of my sexuality that I'll share. I hadn't had intercourse in decades. That's right. Decades. I had an opportunity that I thought might result in intercourse with a guy I'll call Steve. I went to my doctor to get a baseline of STD tests to show I was clean.

I'd been experiencing back pain, and the doctor thought the pain might be related to a prolapsing uterus, which can be common in perimenopausal or menopausal women, or even in runners like myself. Uterine muscles stretched from pregnancy, childbirth, and years of fighting gravity relax to the point where the uterus can be seen in the vagina, or worse, it can descend out of the vagina. The doctor referred me to a rather interesting physical therapist he thought might be able to help. I had no idea what was about to happen.

The therapist specialized in helping women strengthen their pelvic floors, or in simple language, not give birth to their uteruses. And so began one of the most unusual evaluations I had ever experienced. Keep in mind that, as a runner for thirty-five years, I had seen my share of traditional physical therapists who do the usual evaluations of feet, knees, hips, and other appendages. But this PT did a probe of my innards like no other therapist. She measured the degree of prolapse and atrophy of various muscles of the vaginal wall. Her prescription? A dildo. In fact, after taking measurements, she said she would go with a coworker to purchase one at the nearby X-rated adult toy store. What? A health-care professional whose job included buying dildos for patients? And health insurance paid for it?

At the next appointment, she brought in a long, slender, silicone-covered vibrating dildo. Her instructions: "This is not necessarily to get you to the point of climaxing. The goal is for you to have the dildo massage the muscles that have atrophied from not having intercourse all these years. When the muscles tighten, your uterus won't feel like it's about to fall out. The dildo will help stimulate the nerves and encourage blood flow. It's the old use-it-or-lose-it in play here." It all sounded very clinical to me. I don't know if it really worked, but during the time I kept my appointments, I told her that I had an opportunity to have actual sex with a new partner. She immediately looked very concerned and serious. "You're going to need lubricants because it'll be very painful. Your vaginal walls have thinned, and you're not as flexible as you used to be in that part of your body. You'll need to keep doing your slow and fast kegels twice a day."

I stocked up on three different kinds of lubricants, making sure they were vegan, and if possible, organic, of course. When I went to Steve's house where the "activity" was to occur, I secretly slid the lubricants under my pillow. But lo and behold, as the evening unfolded—in fact, as the entire week of lovemaking unfolded—I didn't need a single one of those damn lubricants. Nope, not a one. I returned a couple of them to the pharmacy but left one of them under the pillow as a surprise for Steve, and a reminder of how far (forgive the pun) I had come.

I went back to the physical therapist, not because I needed to, but just to tell her that she was dead wrong. I gushed about how my partner glided in and out of me like a well-vegan-buttered cucumber. My juices gushed and flowed for hours, I gushed. Her response when I bragged that I didn't need the recommended artificial lubricants was "Oh, that's just the newness of the relationship. This too will fade." Spoiler alert to mainstream health-care professionals: It didn't fade. Our relationship prevailed for more than a year, and there were never any sexual problems. It was, and may always remain, the best sex of my life, both emotionally and physically.

Sorting Out the Friends with Benefits

Because we were both vegan, I had so much more in common with Steve than anyone else I'd ever had a relationship with. I know other vegan couples who say that too. I can't ever imagine being that much of a soul mate with someone ever again unless the vegan connection is solid. But therein lies the danger. Because Steve was vegan, it created an illusion of decency and courtesy that, in retrospect, didn't exist. To a woman, a relationship with a vegan guy is so romantic. That set the stage for some pretty powerful delusions.

Another guy I knew told me on our first date that he warned every woman he dated that he had a commitment phobia. He almost seemed proud of it. At least it was clear from the get-go where he stood . . . or where he got laid. But things were murky with Steve. The first time I met him, he recited a long list of women who had been after him in the past year. I joked with him about his harem. "It's not a harem," he said. "Of course it is," I argued cheerfully. I expressed confidence that he was a bright boy and would either figure it out or just enjoy the ride.

We both professed undying friendship because he couldn't use the "R" (relationship) or "L" (love) words. We both spoke of how our mutual passion for veganism fueled our passion in the bedroom. We would both say to each other that it was the best sex we'd ever had, whatever that meant. I felt a deep caring and sharing, a mutuality that resulted in frequent orgasms for both of us and with climaxing at the same time, or close to it. For those in their sixties and beyond, I think that's pretty remarkable and amazing—and, I'm guessing, friggin' rare. I had rarely experienced simultaneous orgasms except in my twenties.

In the prime of our relationship, Steve said once in the heat of the moment, "No matter what happens, let's promise ourselves we'll never settle for anything less than what we have now." He said it almost as a closing argument to himself. In that moment, I knew we both had the best. At the time, I couldn't imagine that he could do better than me. He had told me he liked me better than anyone so far that he'd been with. If he believed I was the best, why would he bail?

I knew that because Steve was (and still is) such a stud, my escapade with him didn't begin or end with me. Unbeknownst to me at the time we met, Steve wasn't at all available to be in a relationship with anyone. He rattled off a litany of women he felt confused about in terms of where he was going in his relationships with them. Part of my reason for getting sucked into the harem I almost mocked during our first conversation was, quite frankly, that I hadn't had intercourse, or even remotely romantic sex, in decades. What little I had gotten felt purely functional, to keep the parts in good working order, and usually the parts I was trying to maintain weren't mine. In other words, my other partners were so focused on their own sexual dysfunctions that I was focused on doing what I could to alleviate that and help them reach orgasm. I had shoved my own sexual pleasure and satisfaction into that shoebox on a shelf, dismissing it as not important. In short, I was lonely.

I knew that Steve's reminders that he wasn't available for a relationship were his way of saying, "It ain't gonna last, so don't get your hopes up or panties in a wad." Did he use me? Yes, he admitted that he liked being seen with me. Ugh. Where are the men who ask questions about your day or want to know what they can do to help you with whatever you need?

This is the ongoing dilemma about the hotly pursued vegan male. Steve fit the role to a T. Of course, I thought if anyone could wow this challenge, that would be me. Even though I talked a good "friends with benefits" lie, I thought I could break that wall down. In the end, the lie was to myself. I thought I could hack it. I was so sex starved that I was content with repeating the mantra "Let's just live in the moment." I truly believed we were doing that. I believed that if it all ended tomorrow, I'd be fine. I'd have the sweet memories of the best sex of my life, and that was that. Oh, that women could borrow a little of the male "I must move on now" mentality.

I thought I had coated my heart in stainless steel. If I could do that, maybe I could handle a relationship that was just in the moment. If I had a nickel for every time I uttered "in the moment" as an affirmation to myself and a directive to Steve (so he could stop stressing about where our non-relationship was or wasn't going), I could make a hefty donation to a favorite animal sanctuary. There was a very brief, intense time when Steve used the "L" word and promised to be more a part of my life. But, as we know, talk is cheap. Actions speak louder than words, and the big "L" never happened.

Alas, I would ultimately lose the battle to stiff competition from women who were needier than I was. Actually, the problem was that I really didn't need anything. I could have used a little love, appreciation, and respect, but I didn't need financial support or someone to save me from a dramatic emotional meltdown. Steve seemed to thrive, as many men do, in a caretaker role. The more rescuing and help a woman needed and the crazier she was (by his own descriptions), the more he was at her side. Apparently the damsel-in-distress fantasy is alive and well.

I definitely had my own identity. But while this sounds a bit old-school, I learned in my TV career that it's often hard for men to cope with strong women. In hindsight, my biggest shortcoming in Steve's eyes was that I was available—and I don't play games.

Steve definitely seemed most connected to and engaged with women who weren't available—either because they lived so far away or they were emotionally wrapped up in a drama he could rescue them from. Men really thrive in that role. By picking women who were about as unavailable as he was, there was no chance any of those relationships would go anywhere. Steve had a long list of complaints about each woman and why she could never be stable, confident, or smart enough to be his soul mate. I had this relationship aced, or so I thought. But like I said, I don't play games well, and I certainly wasn't going to play a role that didn't represent who I am.

Steve and I remain distant friends, as difficult and painful as that's been for me. There have been times in our social-media world when I've wanted to unfriend and disconnect from him. My inner voices tell me, "Whatsamatter with you? You don't need him. He treated you badly. And he's treated others the same way. Dump the guy." Yet I don't pull the plug.

I think it's because what inspired me in his social-media posts ages ago still does. It's the dedication to the cause. The amount of time and thoughtfulness that attracted me in the first place still keeps me interested in what he's thinking and writing. That's what makes it so hard to disconnect, I rationalize. And that's the rub for us vegans. We make exceptions for our partners because they're vegan. We give them a pass because we know how hard it is to find a vegan partner—or even just dependable vegan friends.

One time when I was just about to delete his Facebook friendship, I thought, "I'll copy all our messages from Messenger, just in case those disappear." As I scrolled back a year and a half through the mangroves of passion, despair, and brilliance, I cried one last time, shaking my head in disbelief. How could he have lied? How could he have said all that stuff and reneged? It was truly his loss. I'd like to believe that he had no clue what he was losing. But deep down, he knew.

"He truly didn't deserve me," I self-talked. Rarely do we get to such points in our lives where we feel so deeply hurt. But even if your love is a superstar vegan, it's definitely time to move on if he doesn't love you for exactly who you are. One of these days I may get the courage to unfriend him on Facebook. Part of me wants to try it just to see if he'd even notice; he's so wrapped up in his own drama that it could be months, if ever, before he realizes the breakup was official on social media. It all seems so trivial when you consider how much work needs to be done to save the planet and our own lives. Yet, while it's happening, the pain is real.

One of my friends shared with me some great advice and a beautiful passage she sent to break up with a boyfriend who had ripped her heart out too. It was so gracious and full of love and compassion that only a vegan on the verge of heartbreak could have offered it. She was still primarily thinking of the other person instead of her painful suffering. The following is what she shared with me:

1. I send a golden cord of light from my heart to the person that I am having difficulty with. With my boyfriend, I would send and think, "I send you pure love and light from my heart to yours. For whatever you need. Wholeness in all ways possible." It definitely changed me, and I felt that it made my communication easier and from a place of love (rather than from fear or ego).
2. I acknowledge fully this relationship for the greatest good of all involved. (And I know that *all* includes both me and him). So I can love him fully and be willing to walk away if we don't share a common vision. As I am sure you know, without a common vision, there can be no sustainable relationship.
3. I reminded myself that if this relationship was for my highest and best self, I didn't need to do anything but be my most loving, highest, and best self. If it was a good relationship, it would move further into my life. If it wasn't good for me, then it would move out of my life.
4. Finally, and most importantly, I remembered that the future is based on the now. If the now isn't good, the future won't be. At that time in that now, it wasn't good. I even told my boyfriend this and said, "If you're not available, we need to stop this. I send you love, light, and an abundance of all good things in all dimensions of time—and I release you for whatever pathway you need to take."

She told me, of course, that her heart was breaking when she sent this, but she knew she had to do it. She continued, "All we can ever do is be clear about who we are and the vision we would like to create. We can't bring someone else on board or get them to have our vision. We can hold a space with love and allow what will be—that person will move further into our lives or slowly out."

Another friend, who had observed our non-relationship relationship in action as best as anyone can from afar, had another take on it. She advised, "Take a week to weep and be with good friends, and then allow yourself to get taken out and treated well and make sure that SOB sees it! Remember your self-worth. Remember, he should be begging you to be with him. You're both adults, except he's not stepping up to the plate."

I've read that response from time to time, and it's helped me refocus on why I began this journey in the first place. One line in particular rang so true, as I hope it does for you, male or female: "He should be begging me to be with him."

THE STORY OF JOE

This is such a bizarre story that people told me I had to write it down or sell the movie rights. If you believe in synchronicity, energy that we can't define, or guardian angels, this is one for the record books.

I include it here for several reasons: (1) Just because your guy or gal is vegan doesn't mean that it's a match made in heaven. (2) As more of us become vegan, there's definitely safety in numbers, especially as the vegan community becomes more connected. (3) You can never be too careful or too diligent.

I had called my vegan boyfriend at the time to clarify that we were ending our yearlong relationship. This breakup really was more about him and his personal stressors than anything that had to do with us as a couple. By the end of that phone call I was sure we were done. Really done. There was no doubt. I was a blithering mess.

The only saving grace to the day was that I had a date with a guy that had been arranged through a dating service. Now you might be asking, why would a well-known, otherwise self-confident author hire a dating service? I hate the bar scene. I had moaned to a nonvegan guy friend, "I can't meet any vegan men!" He goes, "What do you mean you can't meet any vegan men! You're on the lecture circuit as a popular vegan author! How can you not meet any vegan men?"

I answered, "What am I supposed to say? Break my professionalism at the end of my talk with 'OK now, if anyone out there knows of a nice vegan guy for me to date, please come up and see me'? I can't do that." He reluctantly agreed, "I guess not." Especially during my career in television, I found that men weren't above confessing that they were going out with me as an "arm piece." The fame of going out with a TV star, or so they thought, was way more important than getting to know me as a person. Deep down, I knew that this latest relationship was the same. Too many comments had surfaced suggesting my lover's interest was more about the eye-candy appeal and hanging out with somebody who had written a book. I just wanted to meet someone and have my identity be anonymous; someone who had no idea who I was, what I did for a living, or even what I looked like. Someone who maybe could support me in a way I had not been supported, maybe ever.

The dating service spent a great deal of time doing in-person interviews and written compatibility surveys. Sadly, I was told, nothing would be asked of me or my prospective partners about dietary preferences or lifestyle values other than religion. They felt that asking whether you wanted your potential partner to show up for dinner every night was more important than knowing what was going to be served on the dinner plate. Even more dismal, I was warned, "Forget about finding anyone in our local database who's vegan. There isn't anyone." OK, I thought. I guess I'm going to have to do my best to sell my date on the many features and benefits of veganism if we were to continue dating. But maybe not on the first date.

The local dating service had called me in advance to let me know that the latest candidate, Joe, had a very good compatibility score and it should be a perfect match. Only one thing didn't fit into my profile, and they wanted to know if I'd make an exception. I only wanted to date guys who were divorced. I didn't want to take a chance on anyone who was still deciding where they stood with an ex.

Apparently Joe was only legally separated from his wife (I'll call her Linda), but they were just a few weeks away from their divorce being accepted by the court. Just a formality, the service said. Was I still interested? They ran down his profile: retired CEO of a wildly successful company. Very fit. Works out every day. Likes dancing, movies, boating, and many of the things I liked. What could possibly go wrong? And if it did, it was just one date.

We went to a posh fish restaurant that had vegan options. We closed down the place five hours later after talking about everything—everything him, that is. It was the reporter in me—I was born asking questions—so the fact that he dominated the conversation didn't seem too out of line. I would have had no problem answering any questions he might have tossed at me, but there weren't very many of them.

At the end of the evening, I looked him squarely in the eyes and said that I had violated my rule of never dating married men because the dating service had said the divorce was imminent, only a formality. "You're not planning to go back to her or anything, are you?" I asked. "Oh no," he insisted without missing a beat. He did say that

Linda became vegan while he was married and perhaps I could get him to go vegan too. Yeah, vegans, especially vegan chefs and authors, get that a lot. I'm so over being anyone's free private chef.

The next morning he called and apologized for asking on such short notice, but there was a national dance competition at the Ritz. Did I want to come? Turned out it was fabulous. The ballroom had a full dance floor and stage lighting, and the floor was surrounded by round tables. We sat in the front row to catch the three-hour show. It was quite something, right out of *Dancing with the Stars*. Interspersed were a few small breaks during which audience members could dance with an instructor or their partner. The whole night felt like a fairy tale, complete with the Cinderella cocktail dress and high-heeled shoes I'd pulled together from a secondhand store for a pittance—because I certainly didn't have dressy clothes like that in my closet anymore. When Joe went to get his car from the valet, I half expected a pumpkin to arrive. At best, it was a great distraction from the breakup I'd just gone through earlier.

When we got back to my condo, which was right on the beach, I asked if he wanted to take a walk. We strolled along the water's edge for about an hour, talking mostly about him, before he drove back home. He texted me several times later that night saying what a great time he'd had. There's a line that I often used to close out many of my TV consumer reports: "If it seems too good to be true, it probably is." I must have thought of that line a dozen times over the weekend, in wonderment, smiling. My smile would soon fade.

Two days later, I had committed to having lunch at an Indian restaurant with our local veg meetup group. A guy across the table from me at lunch mentioned the dance contest and asked, "Did you all hear about it?" Freak coincidence. Me: "I went to that." The woman next to him (second freak coincidence) replies back to me, "With Joe?" Me: "Yes. How did you know?"

Woman: "He's my husband." (Third freak coincidence.) "I went to the contest the next night with another date." She grabbed her phone and scrolled down. "Joe was there that night too. Here's the text he sent to me saying how hot I looked. We're having a date tonight." My mouth dropped open as I saw his text to the wife he was supposedly divorcing and never getting back together with again.

Everyone at the table was as riveted to this discussion as I was, stunned and quickly silent as the story unfolded before us. Like the old game of "telephone," word of what was happening spread down the long rectangular table. Most eyes were staring in our direction.

Everyone seemed incredulous (but mostly me) that this drama was happening live in front of them.

As sad as I was, I was so grateful to have avoided weeks, months, or maybe years of grief. I should have trusted my instincts when I heard Joe plan out loud what our life might be like together—what temperature the house would be set at, what dresses he would buy me, how he might go vegan "this time" if I cooked some vegan meals in his new home that he was still building. (Linda gave me the address. I drove by later and saw the multimillion-dollar monstrosity overlooking the water. It could have been mine. "Let it go," I said silently, chiding my selfish inner voice.)

What were the odds that the universe would place his wife next to me in a group of more than thirty people within hours of my being swept off my feet by her hubby? Those sitting closest to Linda and me at the meetup were the most caught up in the drama. Two of them insisted that we tell them the next chapter as soon as we knew it. They goaded us to play Joe somehow, but neither of us wanted to do that.

Linda told me that she wanted to keep being friends with Joe but that I could have him. She had given up her lucrative career to be a stay-at-home chef and housekeeper in Joe's large house. I told her that she could have Joe all to herself. She assured me she didn't want him and repeated her belief that he had joined the dating service to make her jealous. As you might expect, I never heard from her again and have no idea how their story ended.

But I did text Joe after I had spoken with Linda. At least I had had the presence of mind to take a selfie of Linda and me at the lunch. I sent it to Joe, along with this:

Ellen: "Who woulda thunk? I asked you on my first date if there was any chance of you getting back together with your wife. 'Not at all,' you said. 'Just a formality of paperwork that would happen soon.' The dating service told me the same thing. So I believed you.

"Then you text your wife to tell her how hot she looks a few nights later. And then you go to a movie with her. Who hires a dating service and then goes out with their wife after that? Trying to make her jealous?

"How do I know this? Because I went to one of the very few vegan meetups I ever go to here and happened to sit next to Linda. Someone started talking about the dance competition and, before I knew it, she and I were talking about you! She's lovely. I hope you have a long life together. I was going to tell you in person, but the attached pic should tell you all you need to know. She didn't set it up (as she feared you would think). I just happened to walk into the right place at the right time with some guardian angel watching over me, saving me from heartache. You seemed charming enough; though, as you pointed out, you did almost all the talking.

"I figure, why waste my time? Believe it or not, some women don't give a hoot about money and follow their passion because it's the right thing to do—with or without a man in their life who supports them emotionally. I'm a nice girl with solid midwestern values. I won't be bought by anyone. It was a fun fantasy for a couple of days until I learned the truth. Honesty is what I've built a career on. My unusual energy and life's work are not for sale. We're done."

Joe jumped back immediately to try and convince me that I had it all wrong. But I think I saw his situation much more clearly than he did. I told him he could get back to me once his divorce was final, but not before. It's been a long time since that exchange, and I never heard from him again. Even if he did come back to me with a cleaner slate, trust is an easy thing to lose and, in some cases, impossible to regain. My bad. I should have held my ground with the dating service. Lesson learned. Just because someone is vegan, or vegan friendly, doesn't make them a class act. It doesn't make them relationship or marriage material, as tempting as it might seem.

Linda had shared with me that Joe had been having a long-time affair with another woman. "That's just the way it is," she said. While some people are fine with having multiple relationships at the same time, many of us can't handle that. Better to be alone and content with oneself than be looking for someone else to complete us, right? The old adage that "you must be happy with yourself first before you can truly be happy in a relationship with another" holds true without exception.

I did run into Linda over a year later at a vegan event. We laughed when we recognized each other. I found out on Facebook that Joe did eventually divorce her. Oh well.

THE DARKER SIDE OF A BAD RELATIONSHIP

Dr. Kahn has addressed how having all your parts in working order can make life good both in and out of bed. As he also points out, there are many causes of ED. A variety of issues between men and women may have nothing to do with what comes up, either in that six inches or after sixty years of living.

The older we get, it's common to have regrets and second-guess ourselves, as much as we know deep down we shouldn't. But in wondering how life might have been different in a vegan world, one of the threads woven into my life has been depression and suicide.

One of the most romantic relationships I ever had was with a man I was engaged to, broke up with, then became engaged to again. I'll call him Sam. He always sent me flowers, and we often jet-setted around the Caribbean when he wasn't working long hours building his career. There was something not quite right about Sam that I couldn't pinpoint, and I broke the first engagement off, accepting a TV job in another state. He begged me not to go, and I eventually broke down and decided to stay put.

We ate healthy foods, preparing huge veggie-rich salads every night after work, even though we both ate fish. This was my first experience with a man with erectile dysfunction. He was only twenty-eight. He blamed the problem on everyone and everything in life, mainly his own insecurities. Was it the dysfunctional relationship he had with his parents? Was it his diet?

There were other familial issues in play, but his quick anger got him in trouble when we missed a canceled flight. It was the airline's fault, and he got so mad that security had to be called (and that was back in the days when security was rarely called about anything). What scared me most was that he totally blacked out during the incident and didn't recall any of it. He wasn't willing to get help for this problem, and I wasn't willing to gamble my life on someone with very troubling behavior. I called up the scorned news director, found the job offer was still on the table, and ran.

Sam begged me for the better part of the next year to come back. He even contacted my parents. No one ever made such a play for me as Sam did. But the idea of him going behind my back and trying to reach me through my family didn't sit well with me. My parents made no secret that they thought this up-and-coming businessman was perfect for their daughter. And yet, as always, they deferred to my judgment, delivering their frequent line: "Do what makes you happy."

I googled Sam over the years and saw that he had a very successful career and a beautiful home and had done great work improving the lives of others. In the photos I saw, he had a very long line of gorgeous women on his sleeve. He never had children. I contacted him only once, after I was divorced. It was the world's shortest conversation. He said simply, "Not interested." He eventually did marry an attractive, successful woman, and I thought all was well. That is, until I saw a newspaper article pop up about how he had committed suicide. I was shocked. I couldn't imagine what had precipitated that. Had he still been impotent all those years? Despite his success as we define it in our culture, was it all a cover for those deep-seated insecurities that probably hadn't been resolved and perhaps grew in a perpetual, vicious cycle of personal failure? I could only imagine. I'll never know.

I assumed by the photos I saw of his increased girth that his diet didn't remain as healthy as it was when I knew him. Did the ED and resulting depression get him in the end? Was there anything I could have done? I've asked that a thousand times since I saw the article. Would a vegan diet have cleared out his arteries and the capillaries in his heart and brain to make life better? A vegan diet has been associated with alleviating symptoms of depression. Many studies show that vegans suffer far less from depression, anxiety, stress, and mood swings than meat eaters. If Sam had gone vegan, could his suicide have been averted?

A friend chided me, saying, "Of course there was nothing you could have done. You tried. He rejected you years ago. You were so young when you had your relationship. How could either of you have known what you wanted or that it could have even lasted? If you had married, think of the heartache you would be suffering now." She was right. Our relationship may not have survived. I don't tolerate out-of-control anger very well. But this is one chapter that will always suffer an endless number of unresolved questions.

There's so much research now supporting increased levels of serotonin, a chemical that improves mood, with vegan eating. A 2012 study in *Nutrition Journal* stated that consuming fruits and veggies could effectively increase serotonin levels, which could in turn increase the desire to have sex. People who don't eat any meat tend to be happier and less stressed than those who eat meat. The researchers thought this might be due to arachidonic acid, an omega-6 fatty acid found primarily in animal foods that can cause significant changes in the brain that affect mood.

We definitely need more studies. Although I know of one vegan man who committed suicide, most of the vegan men I have known are happy spirits, at least on the surface. More men than women commit suicide, and people diagnosed with bipolar disorder commit suicide at a rate higher than the general population. It could be argued that many people choose how they leave this earth by adopting lifestyles that cause preventable disease. But I will always wonder about Sam.

It's important for both sexes to be aware of the risk for depression and how that can be helped if a partner transitions to veganism. It provides so many physical and emotional benefits. Stress the positive, but realize it's important not to stifle or redirect feelings. Put problems in perspective. It's so easy to get access to graphic information on the plight of animals or the effects of diet-related diseases, and this can be downright traumatic in and of itself. It's important to be able to compartmentalize this realism, shelve it for the short term, and give ourselves permission to have a good time.

LOOKING AHEAD TO BETTER LOVE DOWN THE ROAD

It can be a rocky road out there in the unpredictable world of relationships, but I wish for you nothing but good karma, bliss, and joy. To the extent you can benefit from my mistakes and experiences, I open my heart widely. No one should experience preventable physical and emotional pain and suffering. Thanks to the courageous vegan doctors and dietitians who share their knowledge and time with us, we know much more about how to achieve health and happiness.

7 vegan aphrodisiacs

by Ellen Jaffe Jones, Beverly Lynn Bennett, and Joel Kahn, MD

PLANTS FOR YOUR PANTS

BY BEVERLY LYNN BENNETT

The word "aphrodisiac" comes from the Greek name Aphrodite, the goddess of love and beauty. This term is applied to foods and drinks that are believed to increase the desire for sex or enhance sexual experience. Throughout history, various herbs, spices, fruits, and vegetables have been called aphrodisiacs simply because of their physical resemblance to female or male genitalia—think figs, cucumbers, and bananas. Other foods have achieved this distinction because of the mental or physical benefits they provide, such as mood elevation, increased blood circulation and muscle control, heightened sexual arousal, or improved stamina and sexual performance. When it comes to aphrodisiacs, much of the information about their benefits is purely anecdotal, but they may be just the thing you need to make you feel more sexual and help you get more going on in the bedroom.

Before veganism was a thing, many of us grew up believing that oysters and other mollusks were perhaps the only passion-inducing foods. Nothing could be further from the truth. Many healthy vegan foods are loaded with sex-enhancing qualities. Since we know that meat clogs the arteries like blocked plumbing, the converse is true. Vegans eat lots of foods rich in nutrients that promote good circulation (such as vitamins A, C, and E, and the mineral potassium), so no supplements are needed.

Following is a list of some of our favorite vegan aphrodisiacs, in addition to the foods shown to promote erectile health that Dr. Kahn mentioned on pages 18–21. One or more of these plant-based foods are used in each of the recipes in this book (pages 93–217).

ALMONDS: This nut is one of the earliest cultivated foods and has been regarded as a symbol of fertility throughout history. In fact, the tradition of having almonds at a wedding began during Roman times—guests would throw the nuts at newlyweds. It's also believed that the smell of almonds incites passion in women.

APPLES: This juicy, sweet fruit is irresistible. Most of us know about Adam and Eve's inability to resist the temptation of "the forbidden fruit" (supposedly an apple) that led to the couple's being expelled from the Garden of Eden. Eating an apple a day may help women to increase vaginal lubrication and improve sexual function and satisfaction.

ARTICHOKES: According to Swedish folklore, women who were feeling a bit neglected in the bedroom would serve artichokes to their lovers to help stimulate their sexual desire and stamina. The French are also fond of artichokes, favoring mostly the inner heart. They incorporate it into many dishes, as they believe it stimulates the genitals of either sex.

ARUGULA: This peppery-tasting leafy green, called rocket in Australia and England, is a delicious addition to salads. Arugula also helps promote good digestion. The Greeks and Romans often associated arugula with the fertility god Priapus, perhaps because the potent amount of vitamins A and C it contains increases the intensity of an orgasm.

ASPARAGUS: This delicious spring vegetable was touted as an aphrodisiac as early as the seventeenth century. Prenuptial dinners in nineteenth-century France often included three courses of asparagus. Asparagus is high in vitamin E, which increases blood and oxygen flow to the genitals, and folic acid, which is said to boost histamine production, which is necessary for both sexes to reach orgasm.

AVOCADOS: The much-beloved avocado boasts a feminine hourglass shape. That said, unripe avocado fruit hangs in pairs much like male genitalia. Avocados are high in omega-3 fatty acids and potassium, as well as vitamin B_6, which is known to increase male hormone production. They're thought to be so effective as aphrodisiacs that Spanish priests used to forbid their parishioners to eat them.

BANANAS: Regarded as a symbol of fertility by Hindus, bananas have an appealing sensual shape that often leads to the desire to ravage the fruit with gusto. They're chock-full of B vitamins and potassium, both of which are needed to produce sex hormones. Additionally, bananas contain the enzyme bromelain, which enhances male libido.

BASIL: This member of the mint family helps promote circulation and is believed to stimulate the sex drive. In Moldovan folklore, a man is destined to fall in love with a woman if he accepts a sprig of basil from her. Basil has a wonderful aroma and is commonly used to make pesto.

BEETS: According to Greek mythology, Aphrodite ate beets to enhance her appeal to others. The Romans believed that they felt more amorous when they consumed either the flesh or juice of beets. This may have to do with beets containing a high amount of boron, a trace mineral that increases the body's sex hormones, and tryptophan, which can promote a feeling of well-being, thereby elevating mood and enhancing sexual arousal.

BERRIES (blackberries, blueberries, cranberries, raspberries, and strawberries): These flavorful morsels are bursting with juice, making them the perfect sweet and healthy treat for nibbling on with your lover. (Or nibbling them off your lover very, very slowly.) The Romans associated strawberries with Venus, the Roman goddess of love, because of their heart-shaped appearance and libido-enhancing properties. Many of the phytochemicals and antioxidants found in berries help to reduce inflammation in the joints. Berries also contain anthocyanins, phytochemicals that give them their rich blue, black, and red colors and that also help to reduce the risk of heart attack. Daily intake of blueberries is associated with helping to prevent Alzheimer's disease. Strawberries contain quercetin, a phytochemical that protects against heart disease.

CARDAMOM: Both the whole cardamom pod and the ground spice (made from the tiny seeds inside the pod) have a sweet, delicate flavor with enticing floral undertones. Some people like to chew on cardamom seeds to freshen their breath. Additionally, cardamom has anti-inflammatory properties that help to increase blood flow. Cardamom is often used to flavor cookies, desserts, and Indian chai tea.

CARROTS: For some people, it may be the phallic shape of carrots that's so appealing; for others, it may be the sweet taste and vibrant hue. Either way, carrots are a must-have in any kitchen, as this versatile vegetable can be used to make a wide range of foods, from beverages and savory dishes to sweet desserts. Carrots are also an excellent source of beta-carotene, which aids hormone production. For guys, carrots can give a boost to sperm production.

CELERY: A bunch of celery has a somewhat phallic form that makes it visually appealing. Also, many people think celery has a scent reminiscent of androstenone (a natural pheromone) and that eating it can stimulate the release of sex hormones.

CHERRIES: Both sweet and sour cherries are packed with many beneficial nutrients, such as folate, iron, magnesium, potassium, and vitamins A, C, and E. They also contain melatonin, a hormone made in the pineal gland that helps to regulate the sleep cycle. Cherries contain several antioxidants that help keep skin radiant and youthful, as well as quercetin, which has antihistamine properties that can come in handy during physical exertion.

CHIA SEEDS: Tiny chia seeds were highly prized by the ancient Aztecs and Mayans and were a staple of their daily diets. Some of the noteworthy benefits of consuming chia seeds include decreased inflammation and joint pain, increased energy and stamina, and enhanced athletic performance—all of which can be beneficial in the bedroom.

CHILES: Whether hot or mild, chiles and ground spices made from them (such as cayenne, chili powder, and paprika) not only add piquant flavor to food, but they also can spice up your love life. Chiles are high in capsaicin, which can increase circulation, pulse rate, and body temperature (often causing a person to perspire), and this mimics arousal or the sexual experience. Additionally, capsaicin is great for reducing pain and inflammation in muscles and joints. Chiles contain substances that signal the brain to release endorphins that enhance overall well-being and improve mood.

CHOCOLATE, CACAO, AND COCOA POWDER: Lusciously rich chocolate is a Valentine's Day staple for a reason. This yummy food contains both anandamide, a psychoactive feel-good chemical, and phenylethylamine, a chemical that releases dopamine in the pleasure centers of the brain and produces feelings of excitement and happiness. Chocolate also contains tryptophan, another happiness-enhancing chemical that the brain needs in order to release serotonin. Consuming the naturally occurring caffeine found in cacao powder, cocoa powder, and chocolate will give you more energy.

CILANTRO AND CORIANDER: Cilantro is a leafy herb, while the seeds of the cilantro plant are called coriander. Both are used prominently in Asian, Indian, Latin American, Mexican, and Middle Eastern cuisines. They have anti-inflammatory, warming, and expectorant properties.

CINNAMON: One of the most commonly used seasonings, cinnamon is often called a warming spice because it stimulates both body temperature and appetite, and for many people, sexual appetite as well. Using cinnamon may help lower your blood pressure and improve mental alertness. Sprinkle some on a plate to help neutralize odors in the kitchen or bedroom. Cinnamon, cloves, ginger, and nutmeg are combined to make pumpkin pie spice, and the scent of pumpkin pie has been documented to increase penile blood flow by 40 percent!

CLOVES: For thousands of years people have been chewing on cloves to help freshen their breath, which definitely doesn't hurt when you're trying to get things going with your sweetheart. Cloves are very aromatic and are often paired with cinnamon or nutmeg in recipes.

COCONUT (fresh and dried), COCONUT MILK, AND COCONUT WATER: The water found inside a coconut has the same amount of electrolytes as blood. Coconut-based products are not only fragrant and delicious but they're also rich in calcium, lauric acid (which boosts immunity), magnesium, potassium, and vitamin C; consuming these nutrients can boost metabolism and blood flow.

COFFEE: The smell of fresh coffee is enough to get some people turned on. A dose of caffeine can boost heart rate and blood flow and increase levels of dopamine (the neurotransmitter associated with the pleasure response in the brain). Although the consumption of coffee in reasonable amounts can be health promoting, drinking too much can cause some people to experience the jitters.

CUCUMBERS: Perhaps it's the cucumber's phallic shape or maybe its aroma, which is believed to increase blood flow to the vagina, that fosters its association with sex. Long-standing rumors about the use of cukes as stand-ins for vibrators has often made them the butt of jokes. Cucumbers contain silica, which keeps skin vibrant and healthy, reduces water retention, and supports the connective tissues that help you stay limber and ready for action.

DATES: According to Ayurvedic teachings, eating dates purifies the blood and increases semen production in men. Dates are extremely sweet, which is why they're often used as a sweetener in recipes by raw foodists and people who want to limit their consumption of processed sugar. Dates can give you an energy boost, which can come in handy during sex.

FENNEL: Fennel has a subtle flavor of licorice or anise. The entire vegetable can be used in cooking. The feathery fronds (which resemble dill) are used as a decorative garnish, the crisp stalks can stand in for celery, the bulb is often thinly sliced or cubed (and eaten raw or cooked), and whole or ground fennel seeds are often used to flavor savory dishes (most notably sausages). Some of the reported benefits of fennel include reduced inflammation, improved circulation and vision, enhanced immunity, a more youthful appearance, and increased vigor.

FIGS: In the biblical story of the Garden of Eden, Adam and Eve used fig leaves to protect their modesty. Figs were also Cleopatra's favorite fruit, and the ancient Greeks associated them with love and fertility. Figs contain high levels of amino acids, antioxidants, and flavonoids that are effective at increasing libido and stamina in both males and females.

GARLIC: This member of the onion family contains allicin, an ingredient that increases blood flow. Both the Hindu and Jain religions believe that garlic not only warms the body but also increases desire. Of course, eating a lot of garlic can cause you to reek of it, so you may want to steer clear of it on a first date.

GINGER: Known as one of the top natural anti-inflammatories, ginger can reduce muscle soreness and increase blood flow to every part of the body. Fresh, dried, candied, and crystallized ginger all can add zest and flavor to beverages, salads and slaws, soups, stir-fries, and other savory and sweet dishes.

GRAPES AND RAISINS: Throughout history, grapes have been a symbol of romance, love, and fertility. The Greek god Dionysus and his

Roman counterpart Bacchus were thought to protect the harvesting of grapes, winemaking, and fertility, and it's said that orgies were held to honor these gods and the rituals that surround them. Newlyweds would be given clusters of grapes, as it was believed their seeds would help bless the couple with many children. In most museums, you'll find cultural artifacts depicting the cultivation of grapes as well as their consumption, including images of people holding or nibbling clusters of grapes or drinking the juice and intoxicating wine that's made from them.

MANGOES: This tantalizing, succulent fruit is believed to increase male libido and virility. In India it's customary to hang mango leaves above the doorway of a honeymooning couple's new home as a fertility charm. Mangoes are an excellent source of vitamin E, which is often affectionately referred to as a sex vitamin because of its reputation for increasing sexual arousal in both men and women.

MINT: The fragrance of mint has long been considered a sexual stimulant because it's refreshing and relaxing to men and women alike. Mint has antiseptic and anti-inflammatory properties and helps to alleviate insomnia and headaches.

MUSHROOMS: Mushrooms are often found hidden in forest foliage, which not only makes them hard to acquire but also adds to their mystique. Some cultures believe that eating mushrooms increases stamina and strength and even longevity. The aroma of mushrooms is often described as earthy, pungent, or funky. They contain high concentrations of the pheromone androstenone, which increases attraction to the opposite sex. Additionally, some people think that mushroom caps resemble the rounded head of a penis.

NUTMEG: Grated nutmeg is highly prized by Hindus because it sweetens the breath. The warming properties of this spice can stimulate sexual appetite as well. Freshly grated nutmeg has the best flavor and aroma, and it pairs nicely with cardamom, cinnamon, cloves, and ginger.

OKRA: In Africa okra was once affectionately referred to as "lady's fingers," and it was believed that eating them would ignite a passion for sex. In India it's thought that oka rejuvenates and activates sexual desire. Okra is rich in B vitamins, folate, magnesium (a natural relaxant), iron, and zinc, all of which help keep the sex organs happy and healthy.

OLIVES AND OLIVE OIL: Plump olives and their fragrant and fruity oil are good sources of monounsaturated and polyunsaturated fats, which aid in blood flow and hormone production. They're both used prominently in Greek, Italian, and Spanish cuisine, as these cultures believe that consuming olives makes men more virile.

PAPAYAS: The lusciously sweet flavor and vibrant color of papaya is quite enticing, and many people believe that the peppery-tasting seeds have contraceptive properties. Papaya is also packed with vitamin A, which helps combat cell aging.

PINE NUTS: In the Middle Ages people believed that eating pine nuts would give them a healthy sex drive. These rich, oily seeds are high in zinc and are delicious when used in pesto and other savory dishes.

PINEAPPLES: At one time pineapple was used as a treatment for impotence. Pineapple is a great source of vitamin C, manganese, and thiamine, as well as bromelain, which can help reduce inflammation resulting from arthritis, sprains, strains, and surgery.

POMEGRANATES: Some people believe the biblical forbidden fruit wasn't an apple but actually a pomegranate. Its crimson seeds are considered to be a symbol of abundance and fertility. Eating pomegranate seeds or drinking pomegranate juice can help lower cortisol levels. It also can increase testosterone production in both men and women, which can heighten sexual desire. Pomegranate has high levels of nitric oxide, a substance that opens up blood vessels, increasing blood flow and genital sensitivity and reducing erectile dysfunction.

PUMPKIN SEEDS: Like many other seeds, tasty green pumpkin seeds are high in energizing zinc. This can be beneficial for keeping the prostate healthy, elevating testosterone levels, and increasing sperm production.

SOY, SOY MILK, TEMPEH, TOFU, AND OTHER SOY PRODUCTS: Soy foods are wonderfully versatile and great sources of plant-based protein, which helps to lower cholesterol levels and blood pressure while boosting circulation. Soy's nutrients have been linked to a reduction in premenstrual syndrome (PMS), and the phytoestrogens (plant estrogens) it contains can help increase vaginal lubrication. The benefits for guys are even better; soy has been found to lower men's risk of prostate cancer (the prostate is a vital gland for keeping everything pumping in the bedroom). Researchers at Kansas State University found that soy protein was just as good as beef for men trying to gain muscle mass, without the heart-attack-inducing cholesterol.

TOMATOES: Tomatoes were once referred to as "love apples" because many people find their tender flesh and juice to be erotic and sensual. Dining on tomatoes before sex may help calm anxiety and improve muscle control, and their natural acidity stimulates blood flow to the lips and mouth.

VANILLA: The intoxicating floral undertones of vanilla are hard to resist. One whiff of vanilla is often all that's needed to get someone in a romantic mood. Vanilla can also mildly stimulate nerve endings, which in turn can make sexual stimulation and sensations even better.

WALNUTS: The omega-3 fatty acids found in walnuts can help ward off cardiovascular disease, aid an erratic heartbeat, and improve blood circulation. Walnuts are high in protein, iron, and zinc, as well as the amino acid arginine. Arginine is converted by the body into nitric oxide, which widens blood vessels and enhances blood flow to the penis.

WINE, BEER, AND OTHER ALCOHOLIC BEVERAGES: Wine is rich in polyphenols and antioxidants (such as resveratrol) that can improve circulation and boost blood flow to the sex organs. Having a glass of wine or another alcoholic beverage can also lower inhibitions and enhance a romantic evening. But keep moderation in mind; too much alcohol can lead to drowsiness or a premature ending to your night's sexual escapades.

HERBS FOR YOUR PANTS

BY JOEL KAHN, MD

You exercise. You eat kale salads, watermelon, pine nuts, and arugula smoothies. And yet you're still hungering for more sexual prowess, duration, and bravado. What can you turn to if you shun expensive prescription drugs like Viagra? Herbs! There's plenty of data and anecdotal evidence showing that using plants for what's in your pants will make your sexual fire burn even brighter. Many of my patients have found that single herbs and adaptogens (plants with healing properties) or combinations of sexually stimulating and supportive plant-based substances can raise their interest and improve their success in the carnal arts. Let's look at some of the most useful plant-based preparations for taking your vegan sex to a higher plane.

Bergamot

Bergamot is a citrus fruit that looks like a lemon and grows on a tree only in the region of southern Italy called Calabria, very close to Sicily. The fruit's pulp has a unique combination of flavonoids, such as bruteridin, melitidin, and naringin. These natural compounds block the same enzyme that statin medications (such as Lipitor) block, without the detrimental side effects. Bergamot has been shown to lower blood sugar, reduce inflammation, improve blood vessel activity, and activate an enzyme system in the same way as the popular diabetic drug metformin.

Does bergamot work in patients? The science says yes, and my experience does too. In a recent trial of seventy-seven individuals with high cholesterol, the participants were treated with a statin medication alone or combined with bergamot. The combination therapy produced the lowest LDL cholesterol and the highest HDL cholesterol. In addition, measures of damage to blood vessels by oxidation were the lowest when bergamot was added. In other studies, the beneficial effects of bergamot on blood sugar levels and body weight were demonstrated, and it was shown that bergamot can help clear nonalcoholic fatty liver disease and a condition known as metabolic syndrome. But what about sex?

When bergamot is combined with other herbal preparations, it has been shown to reverse ED in men with diabetes mellitus. This may be due in part because bergamot supports healthy blood sugar, blood pressure, and blood cholesterol levels. Bergamot's benefits may also be attributable to its powerful antioxidant properties, which improve endothelial function. It can be safely used in women too and produces virtually no side effects. Bergamot is as good as it sounds. It's a supplement I take daily just for the sexual fun of it!

Damiana

Damiana, also known as *Turnera diffusa*, is a low-growing plant with yellow flowers and fragrant leaves. It's native to the subtropical climates of the Caribbean, Central and South America, Mexico, and southern Texas. The leaves and stem are used to make a mild liquor. Damiana has been used as an herbal remedy for centuries. By the time the Spanish crossed the Atlantic, indigenous cultures had been using it for centuries as an aphrodisiac and bladder tonic. Damiana is said to help enhance sexual health. In a study of 108 women with low sexual libido, a preparation including damiana led to greater interest and satisfaction with sex compared to a placebo.

Epimedium

Epimedium comes from the botanical family *Berberidaceae* and derives mainly from China. As an aphrodisiac, it's better known as "horny goat weed." The epimedium plant contains flavonoids that have antioxidant properties and plant-based phytoestrogens that are weak, similar to those found in soy. A particular phytoestrogen, epimedium icariin, increases our friend NO and may also increase testosterone, which would make it an extremely potent aphrodisiac. Epimedium has also been used in the treatment of erectile dysfunction. It may improve the sexual health and performance of women due to the production of NO and subsequent improved flow of blood to the sexual organs, clitoris, and vagina. In a study of men with ED, a compound containing epimedium was superior to a placebo for better sexual performance.

Eurycoma Longifolia (Tongkat Ali)

E. longifolia is a flowering plant commonly known as tongkat ali in Southeast Asia. It grows in Indonesia, Malaysia, and Vietnam, where it's used for medicinal purposes. The root of the plant can be boiled in water and the water consumed as a health tonic and an aphrodisiac. In some cultures the leaves are also used as a source of bioactive compounds. This herb is known to have anti-inflammatory and antioxidant actions that likely improve ED and lead to enhanced sexual performance.

In Western societies, *E. longifolia* is generally known as an aphrodisiac, and there have been a number of scientific studies analyzing its benefits in humans. Of eleven studies done over the last few decades, seven found strong associations between the use of this supplement and improved sexual health and performance. In an evaluation of the research on *E. longifolia* and erectile function, two other studies involving almost 140 men reported significant improvement in measures of erectile performance, particularly in those with the poorest performance to begin with.

L-Arginine

You previously learned about the role of L-arginine (see page 20), an amino acid, as a precursor to NO production, particularly if the enzyme called eNOS (funny that it rhymes with "penis") is functioning efficiently to pump out NO. The discovery of this pathway was part of the research that won the Nobel Prize in Medicine in 1998. There are supplements that have L-arginine alone or in combinations that enhance sexual responsiveness. L-arginine can be combined as L-arginine-HCl (hydrochloric acid), but a particularly interesting form is L-arginine alpha-ketoglutarate. When this form is broken down, glutamine is released, which may be beneficial for gut and brain health as well as be a bonus to boner support. There are dozens of studies on L-arginine and sexual responsiveness with many supportive findings.

There's a single study of patients who suffered a heart attack that didn't favor using L-arginine in high doses. I usually avoid it in patients who have had a recent heart attack, but lower-dose forms, particularly with L-arginine alpha-ketoglutarate, are likely fine. I especially like some L-arginine alpha-ketoglutarate supplements that combine dietary nitrates (red spinach) and polyphenols from apples and grapes that boost the function of eNOS and provide triple-powered support for NO production and sexual performance.

Maca

Maca, technically known as *Lepidium meyenii*, grows in the Andes of Peru. It's cultivated predominantly for its root, which is reported to have powered the Incan empire and its warriors. The powdered root is considered safe to eat and contains glucosinolates similar to those found in cruciferous vegetables, such as broccoli. Maca has been reported in testimonials to increase sexual performance in both men and women, as well as to relieve symptoms of menopause. It's widely available in both powder and capsules and in combination with other substances. There are many scientific references for maca root, including some support that it enhances sexual performance.

Magic Velvet Bean

Yes, I know it sounds like the name of a dancer at a club near an airport, but there *is* a sex-enhancing herb called magic velvet bean. This herb has been used for sexual support, infertility, and nervous disorders. It's also known by its botanical name, *Mucuna pruriens*, which is in the *Fabaceae* family (no relationship to Fabio). It derives from ancient Indian Ayurvedic sources and is a powerful antioxidant that favors healthy arteries. Extracts of the seeds and leaves are available in various preparations combined with other herbs to support successful sexual outcomes. Available data for magic velvet bean shows that it improves sperm motility and possibly fertility (something you may be interested in . . . or perhaps quite the opposite).

There are also reports of it darkening hair and improving measures of Parkinson's disease.

Tribulus

Tribulus is an extract of an herb called *Tribulus terrestris*, which contains many active agents, including steroidal saponins and sterols. There are reports that tribulus compounds help support normal reproductive function and hormone production in both men and women, promote vitality and stamina, support physical endurance, and promote sexual prowess and an overall feeling of well-being. In a rare study of sexual responsiveness in women, tribulus was shown to increase the libido of women who previously had low interest.

Sex-Promoting Herbals as Part of a Vegan Diet

Overall, the best way to preserve and enhance sexual performance is to lead a lifestyle most favorable to artery health. This would include abstaining from smoking; exercising regularly; maintaining normal blood pressure, blood sugar, and blood cholesterol; and achieving an ideal body weight. A whole-foods, plant-based diet will give you many of these benefits. For individuals who already have endothelial dysfunction leading to sexual impairment, the range of herbs described in this chapter, either alone or in various combinations, may support and enhance successful sexual activities. At the end of the day, plants can rock your sexual health, whether eaten in your favorite recipes or taken as supplements.

8 exercises to spice it up

by Ellen Jaffe Jones

Did you think the two hundred calories you burned during that last orgasm was enough for your daily or weekly workout? It might be all that some people need, or want, or can do. But if you want to keep your machine well oiled and optimally functioning, you may want to think about the regular tune-ups that are necessary to keep your parts lasting for a long while and running at peak performance over a lifetime.

When it comes to fitness, I'm a crazed woman by anyone's standards. I watched my aunt die of breast cancer when I was five, and then three more female family members contracted it. I knew exactly what was in store for me if I didn't try to defy my genes and fight to stay in shape. People often ask me what they think is a cutesy question: "What are you running from?" I answer, "Disease." It's that simple. But running or being at the top of your game, whatever that is, takes warm-ups, cooldowns, and maintenance. Athletes don't just run out on the field and start playing.

While veganism can help keep you healthy in so many ways, it isn't a guarantee against all things bad. No matter what you eat, the aging process will thin membranes of the vagina and urethra, and cervical mucus can diminish. But there's much you can do to fight the aging process, so don't give up just yet. One study shows that years of practicing yoga can be very helpful for women entering menopause. Some yoga poses, such as twists, target the adrenal glands and kidneys, producing just enough estrogen to give you an extra edge. The benefits of any exercise will pay off for the rest of your life.

A WORKOUT SPECIFIC FOR SEX?

I wouldn't have thought there was a thing to add to this chapter other than generic advice: stay in shape and eat a healthy, balanced vegan diet, and you'll be good to go. But then the bottom fell out. My bottom, literally. As I describe in chapter 6, a prolapsed uterus can result from the toll gravity and age take on our reproductive parts. However, if your body is in good shape, these unavoidable factors will have less of an impact.

Many newbie vegans who lose weight, recover their health, and enjoy newfound energy after a lifetime of sedentary habits ask me how to start a fitness program. When I wrote the book *Vegan Fitness for Mortals*, I wanted to use my experience as a personal trainer to provide an entry-level plan for whatever sport or activity someone might find appealing.

The same exercises that are perfect for fitness programs are also great for sex. I hadn't really given it serious thought at the time, but when I did later on, I realized that many exercises that are good for keeping in the innards are also good for priming the muscles used in the bedroom. One lover once told me, "I think that running is really paying off in the way you have orgasms and the foreplay beforehand." When you think about it, exercises that maximize the gluteus maximus also maximize all the muscles involved in reaching the summit of that sexual mountaintop. Here's a stunning fact: there are more than six hundred muscles in the body, and when we have sex, we use every single one of them!

With all the running I do, I've no doubt put many physical and massage therapists' children through college in the process of ensuring that all my body parts will continue to function well. Having learned so much about what these professionals recommend (as well as learning from my experience and training), I've developed a routine of exercises that will keep you fit and nimble.

First and foremost, stay in good overall shape the best you can. Keep your aerobic activity at a level that will help you maintain a healthy weight. While some other experts might disagree, I think it can be helpful to include some green tea, coffee, or other source of caffeine to boost your resting metabolism.

Also add some activity that will help you maintain muscle mass, such as weight or resistance training, which is static activity (think bench and leg presses, free weight arm curls, or resistance bands you hold or slip into with your ankles), or dynamic muscle training. You could also include more daily activities that require you to lift.

Exercises to Keep You Happy In and Out of Bed

For each of the warm-ups, dynamic strength training options, and core exercises described in the pages that follow, do each part of the exercise twenty times unless otherwise indicated.

WARM-UPS

These warm-up exercises are important to do before you begin any activity that's strenuous enough to work up a sweat, such as running, biking, or other cardio. Take a few minutes to do a light workout—such as a jog, brisk walk, or brief bike ride—before you attempt these warm-ups. Even with these initial stretches, it's important to not start out with cold muscles.

You don't have to do all these exercises the first time; try a few and see how it goes. You may reach a point where they become second nature to you, and it's easy to remember them. You'll look forward to doing them to feel optimally warmed up before your workout and to stretch tired muscles after your workout. The goal is to get your blood flowing into the larger muscles, including your heart, so that all your muscles will get the additional oxygen they need to perform well during exercise and recover well afterward.

CIRCLE ROTATIONS: Rotate both feet at the ankles, first in one direction, then the other. Make circles in the air with your feet, swinging below the knees in both directions. Circle the hips in both directions. Circle the shoulders to the front, then to the back.

FOOT STRENGTHENERS: Take steps on your heels, then steps on your toes. Step with your toes pointed in, then with the toes pointed out.

SKIPPING: Skip backward, then forward. While skipping forward, make big arm circles, then repeat with small arm circles. Rest for a moment. Skip forward again, but this time clap your hands high overhead while your right leg is lifted, then underneath the left leg when it's lifted. Repeat, switching legs.

SIDE SLIDES: Hop to the side, going each direction.

CARIOCA OR TWISTING HIPS: Step the right leg up over the left leg, then the left leg back over the right leg. Give your hips a good swing while you're doing this. If you're in good shape, bring each knee as close to your chest as you can.

HIGH KNEES AND BUTT KICKS: Jog slowly, raising your knees as high as you can, then kick your feet back as if you're trying to kick your butt.

DYNAMIC STRENGTH TRAINING

Dynamic strength training uses force, sometimes explosive force, to build muscles. Activities such as walking lunges, skipping with arm circles, and pogo hops will do the trick. The faster you work out, the harder your heart will work. Some people are able to add weights to an aerobic workout, but to avoid injury and burnout, separate the types of workouts you do to ensure you can accomplish your goals.

LUNGES: Bring your arms to shoulder height, then bend them at the elbow with the hands up. (This is the classic cactus position in yoga.) Step forward, bending the knee until the leg below the knee is perpendicular to the ground. Twist right. Then repeat with the left leg, rotating left. Repeat, but this time when you step forward with the right leg, twist left; step forward with the left leg and twist right. Be sure to maintain your arm position as you move.

MONSTER WALK: Bring your arms to the classic cactus position, as for the lunges. With each step, raise your knee and try to touch it to your elbow on the same side. Don't overstretch.

PICK BLUEBERRIES: Take three steps. On the third step, flex your forward foot and lean over at the waist with both arms and palms forward, as if scooping berries or shells off the ground. Stand and repeat, flexing the other foot this time.

OVER AND UNDER THE FENCE: Imagine a barbed wire fence. Going to the right side, step over it sideways, then slide under it sideways. (Crouch down and keep your head low and your back straight so you don't get "snagged" on that imaginary barbed wire!) Repeat on the other side.

HAMSTRING OR TIN SOLDIER WALK: Raise your leg straight and touch it with the opposite hand. Repeat on the other side.

JUMPING JACKS: Do these slowly enough to land flat-footed.

SEAL JACKS: These are like jumping jacks, but instead of bringing your arms overhead, bring them in front of you with your palms together. Be sure to land flat-footed.

GATE SWINGS: Jump your feet out, shoulder-width apart, with your toes and knees pointed out; press your knees open with your hands.

POGO HOPS: Hop quickly a few inches off the ground with your knees straight and arms at your sides. Repeat, but try to jump a little higher.

LEG LIFTS: If you're warming up before aerobic exercise, such as with running or biking, do leg lifts while holding on to a pole for support. Swing each leg out to the side with your foot flexed. Next, turn sideways to the pole and swing each leg out straight in front, and then swing each leg as far as you can to the back.

CORE EXERCISES

Exercise gurus used to think that spot training alone would allow you to get the shapely body you want, but we now know this isn't true. However, developing core strength by focusing on the abdomen, lower back, and pelvis is not only key for athletic performance, but it's also critical for maintaining the muscles that are used in achieving an orgasm or the foreplay leading up to it.

WINDSHIELD WIPERS: Lie on your back, bend your knees to make a right angle, and drop them to the left, almost (but not quite) touching the floor. Lift your knees and drop them to the right. Dropping slowly will work those abs better than dropping them quickly. Alternate side to side with control, ten times on each side.

SCISSORS: Lie on your back and raise your legs until they're perpendicular to the floor. Keeping your legs straight, scissor them up and down slowly, until they almost (but not quite) touch the floor. Scissor the legs back up until your legs are perpendicular to the floor again. Repeat ten times. Finally, do a horizontal scissors by criss-crossing the legs over each other, dropping and lowering as before. Repeat ten times.

HEEL–TOE: Lie on your back and raise your legs until they're perpendicular to the floor. Bend your knees so your shins are parallel to floor. Using one leg at a time, touch your toes to the floor, then your heel. Repeat three times.

BOAT HOLD: Lie on your back and raise your legs until they're perpendicular to the floor. Bend your knees so your shins are parallel to the floor. Curl up, bringing your nose as close to your knees as you can with your arms straight along your legs and your palms facing up. Hold for three seconds, then lie back on the floor. Repeat this five to ten times (or until you can't do any more!).

TABLETOP CRUNCH: Lie on your back and raise your legs until they're perpendicular to the floor. Keep your feet flexed and your arms at your sides, palms down. Focus on raising your lower back and legs into the air so most of the movement is being propelled by your abs, not your legs. Lower slowly; repeat ten times.

BABY CRUNCHES: In order for these to be effective, it's important to go slowly and follow all these instructions carefully so you'll work the right muscles. Lie on your back and raise your legs until they're perpendicular to the floor. Bend your knees, so your shins are parallel to floor. Put your hands behind your head with your fingertips, just cupping your head—not for support but for proper alignment. Keep looking up at the ceiling, not at your knees. Raise your torso from the waist only an inch or two. Focus on this small movement without moving anything else.

PLANK: A plank is a push-up that you hold. You can do planks with straight arms, but if your wrists aren't up for the party, you can do them by balancing on your forearms. In either case, make sure your arms or elbows are directly below your shoulders. Your legs will extend back straight with your toes bent. Keep your body in one straight line—no butt in the air or sagging tummy! Try to hold this for at least thirty seconds, then challenge yourself to hold it longer as you get stronger.

CAT–COW: On your hands and knees (the classic tabletop yoga position), inhale, allowing air to fill your lungs as your midsection sags down like a cow's. On the exhale, arch your body up like a cat. Repeat this movement ten times while following your breath.

FIRE HYDRANT: On your hands and knees, lift one bent leg as if you were a dog peeing on a hydrant. Extend the leg straight to the side, bring it back to the bent position, and then down to the floor. Repeat on the opposite side. Do on both sides ten times.

TABLETOP KICKS: On your hands and knees, extend one leg straight behind you, look back at your foot, and swing that foot sideways toward your waist. Bring it back straight behind you, and repeat ten times. Switch to the other side for another set of ten repetitions.

SEX-SPECIFIC MUSCLE EXERCISES

Since you read my story on page 51 about going to a pelvic physical therapist, you might be wondering what those exercises were about. They're actually good for both men and women. If you're a woman, you'll want to keep your pelvic floor tight enough to support your internal organs. (Women who've had natural childbirth may need to work on this a little more than women who haven't.) Men, if you value your prostate, urethra, sphincters, and the other muscles that control the flow of your lower body bodily fluids, don't pass these up.

KEGELS: Alternate between drawing up your pelvic floor quickly and holding it. Work up to doing one hundred fast kegels. Begin holding the kegels for ten seconds, then work up to holding for twenty, then thirty seconds. Release your muscles for the same amount of time that you held them.

BRIDGES: Lie on your back with your knees bent and feet on the floor. Push your butt up until your body is in a straight line all the way from your bent knees to your chest. If you're able to, raise your body down to your shoulders, but be sure to keep your body straight. Hold for twenty to thirty seconds, then slowly lower. Barely touch the ground, then come back up and hold again. Start by doing ten of these, then work up to thirty if you can.

ONE-LEGGED BRIDGES: Rise up as if you were a bridge (or as if you were doing the yoga bridge pose), then lift and straighten one leg. Keep breathing, hold for ten seconds, then lower your foot to the floor, and repeat with the opposite leg. Do both legs ten times.

BELLY-PRESS CLOCK: Lie on your back with your knees bent and feet on the floor. Put an index finger right below your belly button, and imagine this is noon on a clock. Raise your belly, pressing into the finger, and hold for ten seconds. Move your finger to where three would be on a clock. Raise your belly again, and hold for ten seconds. Do the same at the six and nine o'clock positions. Repeat each rotation twenty to thirty times.

SHEET/TOWEL CRUNCH: Prepare to do a baby crunch as described on page 83. Wrap a long beach towel or bedsheet around your back at the waist, and twist it comfortably at the belly button. As you crunch up, push into and resist the towel, feeling the muscles around your waist. Repeat ten to thirty times.

FLEXIBILITY PAYS IN BED

The best prevention against injury and stiffness (of the wrong kind) in bed is to be healthfully flexible. The following exercises are cooldowns and stretches I use after running, but many of them are adaptations of yoga poses and are good for whatever stiffness ails you. If flexibility exercises are new to you, start slowly, pick a few that seem manageable, and build from there.

Standing Stretches

CALF STRETCH: With straight arms, place both palms against a wall. Lean forward with one knee bent and the other leg straight behind you. Use your hands to press against the wall until you can feel a stretch in the calf of the extended leg all the way down to your heel. If you have trouble feeling this stretch, turn your back foot so the toes are pointed in slightly and the heel is out (pigeon-toed) to intensify the stretch. Hold for twenty to thirty seconds. Repeat with the other leg.

HAMSTRING STRETCH: Find an object about one foot high and flex one foot up against it. Gently lean forward from the waist as far as you comfortably can. Hold for twenty to thirty seconds, then straighten up, and repeat twice. Switch legs and repeat.

QUAD STRETCH: Balance on your left foot with your left hand against a wall. Bend your right knee and grab your right ankle with your right hand. Squeeze your right heel against your butt and straighten up tall until you can feel the thigh muscles of your right leg stretching. The key to feeling this one is squeezing your glutes tight. Hold for twenty to thirty seconds. Switch to the other leg and repeat. You can repeat this exercise one or two more times per leg. Be careful not to torque or stretch the knee too hard.

LOWER BACK STRETCH: Standing up straight, bring your arms out to your sides with your palms up; inhale and touch your palms overhead. Twist your hands so your palms are facing outward, keep your arms straight, and fold forward as far as you comfortably can, letting your arms fall to your sides as you fold. Allow your arms and body to rest bent over like a rag doll. You can hold on to your elbows or let your arms sway from side to side for thirty to sixty seconds. Stand up slowly and repeat.

GROIN STRETCH: With your legs shoulder-width apart and your knees unlocked, grab your elbows and lean over as far as you can without discomfort. Hang there like a rag doll for twenty to thirty seconds until you feel the upper inner thigh stretch. Release your arms, then lean to the left side, bending your left knee slightly and pressing your left elbow against your inner left thigh. Repeat on the right side.

DOWNWARD DOG: Bend from the waist, place both hands on the ground so your body is in a pyramid with your butt in the air, and step your feet back as far you can. Press into your heels. You can "walk the dog" by pushing on your hands in opposition to your feet for about thirty seconds, trying to get each heel in succession to touch the ground.

PIDGEON: Starting from downward dog, bend your right leg. Lower your right knee to the ground just to the inside of your right hand. Bring your right foot as close to your left hand as you can. (Depending on your flexibility, your right foot may end up closer to your left hip than your left hand.) Keeping your left leg straight behind you, gently lower down on your right hip as far as you can. Put a folded blanket under your right hip if needed for comfort. Stay upright with your hips squared; avoid leaning left. Stay there for twenty to thirty seconds. If you're very flexible, bring your weight down on both hips and bend forward until your forehead reaches the ground. Lift yourself up and repeat on the left side.

Stretches from the Ground

BUTTERFLY: Sit on the ground, place the soles of your feet together, and allow your knees to drop open. Grab your toes with your hands and sit up straight. Hold for twenty to thirty seconds; repeat for a total of ten times.

FIGURE FOUR OR THREAD THE NEEDLE: Lying on your back, raise your left leg so that it's straight up in the air. You can either point or flex your foot. Bend your right leg and place the outside of the right ankle just below your left knee. Use your right elbow to press against the inside of your right thigh to stretch your hip flexor. Repeat on the other side. Hold for twenty to thirty seconds; switch legs and repeat on the other side.

NEED SOME VISUAL SUPPORT?

I have videos on my YouTube channel showing the most important exercises I do before I run, as well as the cooldown exercises and stretches I do after I run. They've kept me injury-free through forty-plus years of running and being a gym rat. I may not do them all every time I run, but I try to.

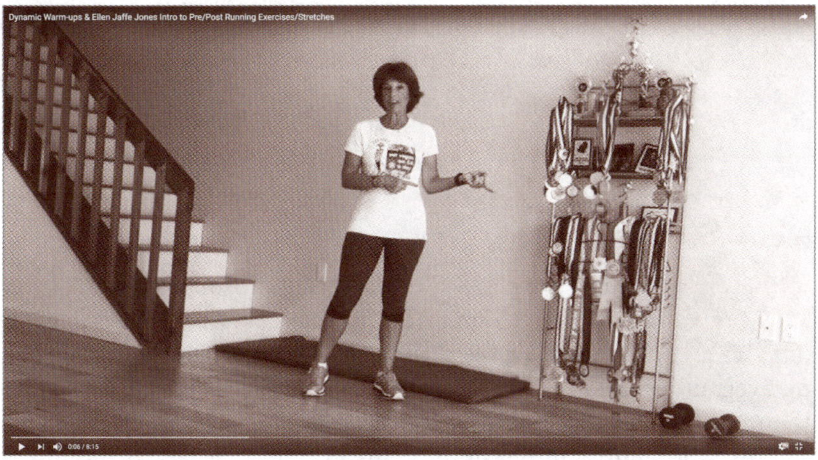

youtube.com/watch?v=KqgWJmRwlHU

9 vegan sex toys and products

BEING MISSION CONSISTENT

by Ellen Jaffe Jones

It was a gorgeous Florida spring morning, and my lover and I were having a leisurely breakfast at a popular restaurant after I had run a 10K race, when we almost lost our vegan cookies. A large truck pulled out of the parking lot onto the main road, and a painting on the side of the truck advertised a sex-toy store with a rather graphic illustration that got the attention of everyone in the restaurant. I immediately googled the name of the store, and much to our delight, we found we were only a few minutes away. We had to check it out.

Neither my lover nor I had been to such a store, and I think we both believed we might find something we couldn't do without. My lover came to veganism for health reasons and had only recently begun to get in touch with the animal welfare problems that are so pervasive around the globe. It seems like you can't go anywhere to escape them. We were horrified to see how many sex toys had real animal fur and skins. (I had no idea the need for vegan sex toys was so important!)

The saleswoman was quite enthusiastic, so I put on my investigative reporter's hat and played totally dumb. I asked her to show me everything, feigning delight and enthusiasm, and inquired whether I could take photos, mainly to help me remember all that I saw. When I asked about the fur, she showed me hunks of animal fur hanging in strips from the wall and responded, "Oh, I know. I hate this. Most of these are from China. They're the worst offenders. There's no regulation." (It's estimated that China makes 70 percent of the world's sex toys.) The employee, almost embarrassed now, showed me several bunny ears that were made from real bunnies. Assorted feather boas and other body decorations, such as nipple covers, included feathers too. I began to envision how animal activists could expand their protests from puppy mills, circuses, and animal captivity venues to sex-toy stores.

When I got back home, I started digging into whatever I could find out about sex toys and was amazed to find a *Forbes* magazine article titled "How The 'Niche' Sex Toy Market Grew into an Unstoppable $15B Industry." The article reported that the sex-toy industry has projected that it will surpass $50 billion in sales by 2020. Just how much of that money is made off the backs of animals? It was difficult for me to judge from the one store I visited, as toys that looked real were fake and some that looked fake were not. I think, for the most part, if you touch the material you can tell whether it's actual animal skin. If there's any good news, it would be that there were far more products that weren't leather, probably because man-made materials are far cheaper. As that's the case with leather shoes and jackets, so it goes for the kinky leather shirts, tops, straps, and any other wearables and props. Faux leather is way cheaper than the real thing now. Feathers are quite another story. With their vivid, intense colors, peacock feathers are pretty easy to spot; they're often used in nipple covers or pasties. Other types of feathers aren't as easy to identify.

You may be a persnickety shopper at Whole Foods, and you may be insistent that your investments are mission consistent by not having companies in your portfolio that test on animals. But are you equally particular when it comes to your bottom orifices? Shoppers don't often consider some of the nasty ingredients that can be found in dildos, vibrators, and lubricants. Some lubricants actually have silicone in them. They largely go unregulated, even the products known as edibles. (For my money, placing dates, grapes, and berries in strategic body locations is a much safer and cheaper way to go.)

One of the biggest problems for the sex-toy industry is the popularity of items made from polyvinyl chloride (PVC). The same PVC formulation that's used in plumbing pipes would be too uncomfortable in a sex toy, so the industry softens the plastic with another controversial chemical, phthalate. Phthalates are particularly cheap and easy to work with. However, studies have shown that exposure to phthalates can cause cancer, and minute levels have been linked to sperm damage. A German study in 2000 found ten dangerous chemicals off-gassed in certain sex toys in Europe. Compounding the problem is that substances containing phthalates can deteriorate over time; when they do, phthalates will be readily absorbed by the body. Not good for a warm, moist vagina. The United States, Europe, Canada, and Japan tightly control the use of phthalates in children's toys but not so much when it comes to products for adults. Some companies have become proactive by not offering products with phthalate; others recommend using a condom with a sex toy.

Whether you want to be sticking silicone and PVC plastic up your vagina is your call. But if you don't, there's a variety of organic products you can choose from. You may have to search for a lubricant that's both vegan and chemical-free, but they do exist. (They might be labeled "fusion of water and coconut oil.") See the resources on page 221.

The safest sex is practiced with condoms, but not all condoms are vegan. In fact, most aren't. Some are even made using casein, a form of cow's milk protein. Others are made from lamb intestines. Major ew! There are nitrile condoms intended to be worn inside the vagina or anus. In case you're wondering what nitrile is made of (because substitutions for harmful chemicals are often worse than the offending ingredient), nitrile rubber is a synthetic copolymer of acrylonitrile (ACN) and butadiene. It's also known as Buna-N, Perbunan, acrylonitrile butadiene rubber, and NBR, with trade names that include Nipol, Krynac, and Europrene. It can be a suitable substitute for anyone with a latex allergy, but not much is known yet about its effects.

TO BOND OR NOT

I'm totally with vegan feminists and others who care about the objectification of women as well as animals. Personally, I'm not into bondage, collars, BDSM, or any other behaviors that exploit women or men—even in fantasy. Just because people are vegan or own a vegan business doesn't automatically mean they align with all your values. The sex-toy industry is huge and appeals to individuals with a wide range of interests, many of which are considered over the top by some people. But thanks to popular media, such as the Fifty Shades erotic romance series by E. L. James, and a prevalent sense that anything goes, the popularization of sexual role playing flourishes.

Many vegans would find bondage fantasies revolting and not worthy of additional consideration. However, people do go there, and that's just the way it is. To those individuals I say, if you're going to buy bondage toys anyway, please go vegan—for the sake of your health, the planet, the animals, and your partner.

10 vegan sex recipes

by Beverly Lynn Bennett

As the vegan movement grows, more opinions arise about the healthiest dietary approaches. Among the most controversial topics has been whether to include oils or high-fat foods. Doctors who encourage low-fat, plant-based eating generally contend that added fats and oils should be avoided for heart health, especially by people who already have heart-related health concerns. Other doctors aren't as quick to swear off nuts and seeds and their oils, acknowledging that consuming a tablespoon or two of nuts, seeds, or oil on occasion won't result in an instant heart attack and may provide essential healthy fats. Including some higher-fat foods could also help more people stick with a vegan diet.

Healthier fats, such as those found in avocados and flaxseed oil, provide essential fatty acids that our bodies need. But if you have any concerns, get baseline blood tests and check with your doctor to ensure that your heart is healthy and these foods won't be a problem for you. Vegan athletes often require the additional calories and satiation that nuts and seeds provide. For some people, though, just looking at a nut can cause weight gain. Nuts are not only calorie dense, but they also are high in fat, so they should be among the first foods to cut back on or cut out completely if you're trying to slim down. The following guidelines are what I generally adhere to: What did Mother Nature intend for us to eat? How did our ancient ancestors eat?

This major disagreement in the vegan community isn't likely to go away anytime soon, so follow what feels right to you for your own body. If you want to decrease the oils or high-fat ingredients in the recipes that follow, knock yourself out, but be aware that the intended outcome of the recipe will change. If you're okay with including higher-fat ingredients, then go for it. We've tried to walk a diplomatic line and follow the latest scientific guidelines as best we can. As with anything, however, we know we'll offend a few people. But don't let that bend you out of shape, unless, of course, you're practicing your vegan sex positions.

recipes

morning quickies

Most people lead busy lives and have many commitments to juggle, so getting moving in the morning can sometimes be a struggle—especially after a night of passion or an early morning quickie. If you're running short on time, regardless of the reason, you'll need a fast fix to fuel up for the day. The speedy beverages, smoothies, fruit-based bowls, and breakfast sandwiches in this section will help get your day off to a great start. You might even have the time and stamina to squeeze in another quickie before you head out the door!

chai tea for two

makes 2 servings

India is famous for its delicious and comforting chai, which is made by brewing black tea with chai masala, an aromatic blend of warming spices. The flavorful tea is then strained, blended with milk, and lightly sweetened. Packaged chai tea is readily available at most supermarkets and natural food stores.

1½ cups water
2 chai tea bags
1 cup almond milk, coconut milk beverage, or other nondairy milk
1½ tablespoons coconut sugar, agave nectar, or other sweetener
1 teaspoon vanilla extract

1. Put the water and tea bags in a small saucepan. Bring to a boil over high heat. Remove from the heat and let steep for 5 minutes. Remove and discard the tea bags.
2. While the tea is steeping, put the milk and sugar in a medium saucepan and warm over medium heat, stirring occasionally, until the milk is steaming and bubbles appear on the surface.
3. Remove from the heat and stir in the vanilla extract. Add the chai tea and whisk until frothy. Serve immediately.

ICED CHAI LATTÉ: After combining the brewed tea with the sweetened milk, let the mixture cool completely. Serve over ice.

Per serving: 55 calories, 1 g protein, 1 g fat (0 g sat), 10 g carbs, 75 mg sodium, 225 mg calcium, 1 g fiber

arousing avocado smoothie

makes 2 servings

This libido-boosting smoothie features fruits and veggies, such as banana, cucumber, and celery, that evoke male genitalia, along with sensual dates and avocado, which the Aztecs affectionately called a "testicle tree" (since the fruit hangs in pairs). Stamina-enhancing chia seeds put this beverage over the top. You might just have to call in late for work, you naughty thing, you.

2 cups baby spinach, kale, or other leafy greens, stemmed and lightly packed
1 cup coconut water or water
1 banana, broken into pieces
1 avocado, diced
2/3 cup diced cucumber
1 large stalk celery, sliced
½ cup ice cubes
¼ cup fresh mint or basil leaves, lightly packed
¼ cup raw pistachios
3 pitted soft dates
Juice of ½ lemon (ABOUT 2 TABLESPOONS)
2 teaspoons chia seeds

Put all the ingredients in a blender and process until smooth. Scrape down the container with a silicone spatula and process for 15 seconds longer. Serve immediately.

turn-ons For an energizing boost, replace the coconut water with 1 cup of cold green tea.

Per serving: 465 calories, 10 g protein, 28 g fat (5 g sat), 53 g carbs, 278 mg sodium, 188 mg calcium, 22 g fiber

mango lassi

makes 2 servings

This yogurt-based drink originated in India. It may be either sweet or salty and is traditionally flavored with spices and sometimes fruit. A lassi provides a cooling effect that helps counter the heat of spicy dishes—unless that "spicy dish" happens to be you! This version is slightly sweet, creamy, and refreshing.

- 1½ cups coconut milk beverage or other nondairy milk
- 1 mango, peeled, pitted, and diced
- 1 container (6 OUNCES) plain or vanilla nondairy yogurt
- 1 tablespoon agave nectar or coconut sugar, or 2 pitted soft dates (PREFERABLY MEDJOOL)
- 1 teaspoon rose water (OPTIONAL)
- ½ teaspoon ground cardamom
- Finely chopped pistachios or almonds

1. Put the milk, mango, yogurt, agave nectar, optional rose water, and cardamom in a blender and process until smooth. Scrape down the container with a silcone spatula and process for 15 seconds longer.
2. Serve immediately, straight up or over ice. Garnish with pistachios.

Per serving: 227 calories, 6 g protein, 5 g fat (1 g sat), 44 g carbs, 122 mg sodium, 528 mg calcium, 5 g fiber
Note: Analysis doesn't include pistachios to garnish.

dutch apple pie smoothie

makes 2 servings

Apples, rolled oats, walnuts, flaxseeds, and spices are blended to perfection. One sip of this love potion will woo your taste buds into thinking you've splurged on Dutch apple pie for breakfast.

- ⅔ cup old-fashioned rolled oats
- ¼ cup raw walnuts
- 2 teaspoons flaxseeds
- 1 cup water or coconut water
- 1 cup plain or vanilla almond milk or other nondairy milk
- 2 medium apples, coarsely chopped
- 4 pitted soft dates
- 1½ teaspoons vanilla extract
- 1 teaspoon ground cinnamon
- ¼ teaspoon ground nutmeg

1. Put the oats, walnuts, and flaxseeds in a blender and process until very finely ground, about 30 seconds.
2. Add the water, milk, apples, dates, vanilla extract, cinnamon, and nutmeg and process until smooth. Scrape down the container with a silicone spatula and process for 15 seconds longer. Serve immediately.

Per serving: 350 calories, 8 g protein, 13 g fat (1 g sat), 56 g carbs, 79 mg sodium, 262 mg calcium, 11 g fiber

spicy bahama mama smoothie

makes 2 servings

Inspired by the popular rum-based cocktail of the same name, this nonalcoholic smoothie is made with a variety of tropical fruits, coconut milk, and orange juice, along with jalapeño chile and ginger to tingle your tongue and excite your senses.

1½ cups fresh or frozen papaya chunks
1½ cups fresh, canned, or frozen pineapple chunks or tidbits
1 mango, peeled, pitted, and diced
1 cup plain or vanilla coconut milk beverage
½ cup fresh or frozen pitted cherries, or ¼ cup pomegranate seeds
Juice of 1 lime (ABOUT 2 TABLESPOONS)
½ small jalapeño chile, seeded
1 (1-INCH) **piece fresh ginger, thinly sliced**

Put all the ingredients in a blender and process until smooth. Scrape down the container with a silicone spatula and process for 15 seconds longer. Serve immediately.

turn-ons Replace any of the fruits in the recipe with the tropical fruits you most prefer, such as dragon fruit, guava, passion fruit (a favorite, of course), or star fruit. If you like, add one or two shots of light rum or coconut rum.

SPICY BAHAMA MAMA BREAKFAST BOWLS: Put only half of the mango in the smoothie and process as directed. Pour into two bowls and top with the remaining mango, 1 peeled and sliced kiwi, and 2 tablespoons of pomegranate seeds or dried goji berries. Serve immediately.

Per serving: 250 calories, 4 g protein, 3 g fat (0.3 g sat), 60 g carbs, 88 mg sodium, 288 mg calcium, 8 g fiber

mexican hot-chocolate smoothie

makes 2 servings

The Mayan and Aztec Indians of Mexico were among the first civilizations to cultivate cacao trees and enjoy chocolate-flavored beverages, a very smart concept! Chocolate gets right to the heart of sexual pleasure by increasing the brain's level of serotonin, the feel-good chemical. This smoothie tastes like chilled hot chocolate. It will rev you up from the inside out.

2 cups plain, vanilla, or chocolate almond milk or other nondairy milk

½ cup ice cubes, or ½ banana, broken into pieces

3 tablespoons cacao powder or unsweetened cocoa powder

2 tablespoons light brown sugar or coconut sugar

1 teaspoon vanilla extract

¾ teaspoon ground cinnamon

⅛ teaspoon cayenne

Put all the ingredients in a blender and process until smooth. Scrape down the container with a silicone spatula and process for 15 seconds longer. Serve immediately.

MACA-MOCHACCINO SMOOTHIE: Replace 1 cup of the almond milk with 1 cup of cold coffee. Decrease the cinnamon to ¼ teaspoon. Omit the cayenne and add 2 tablespoons of maca powder.

Per serving: 91 calories, 3 g protein, 4 g fat (1 g sat), 15 g carbs, 155 mg sodium, 477 mg calcium, 4 g fiber

ambrosia

makes 2 servings

According to Greek mythology, ambrosia was the food of the gods, and if eaten regularly, it would bestow longevity or immortality upon those who consumed it. This refreshing fruit salad is satisfying but light, so it won't weigh you down if you decide to schedule some late-morning action.

2 oranges, or 1 navel orange and 1 blood orange, peeled

1 banana, cut into 1-inch slices

½ cup fresh, canned, or frozen pineapple chunks or tidbits

1 tablespoon agave nectar

¼ cup pomegranate seeds

2 tablespoons unsweetened shredded dried coconut

1 Cut the oranges into segments over a medium bowl to catch the juices and drop the segments into the bowl.

2 Add the banana, pineapple, and agave nectar and gently stir to combine. Scatter the pomegranate seeds and coconut over the top. Serve immediately.

Per serving: 295 calories, 4 g protein, 10 g fat (8 g sat), 55 g carbs, 6 mg sodium, 85 mg calcium, 10 g fiber

passion fruit breakfast bowls

makes 2 servings

Rather than being sipped from a glass, a smoothie bowl is eaten with a spoon. Get your partner relaxed and in the mood by dishing up this ravishing breakfast. It's as irresistible as you are! Among other luscious ingredients, it contains passion fruit, known for its intoxicating flavor and chill-pill properties.

1 mango, peeled, pitted, and diced
1 cup fresh, canned, or frozen pineapple chunks or tidbits
1 frozen banana, broken into pieces
½ cup coconut water or plain nondairy milk
1 passion fruit
1 kiwi, peeled, quartered lengthwise, and thinly sliced
2 tablespoons dried goji berries

1. Put half the mango and all the pineapple, banana, and coconut water in a blender and process until smooth. Scrape down the container with a silicone spatula and process for 15 seconds longer.
2. Evenly divide the blended mixture between two bowls. Cut the passion fruit in half, scoop half the seeds into each bowl, and then swirl the seeds into the mixture.
3. Top with the remaining mango, kiwi, and goji berries. Serve immediately.

Per serving: 278 calories, 4 g protein, 2 g fat (0.4 g sat), 68 g carbs, 70 mg sodium, 63 mg calcium, 9 g fiber

pistachio, dried fruit, and yogurt delight

makes 2 servings

Shrikhand is a traditional yogurt-based sweet that hails from India's western states of Maharashtra and Gujarat. In this version, powdered sugar is pulverized with cardamom and saffron threads, which both tint and flavor the yogurt. The yogurt is then blended and garnished with chopped figs and dates. Crunchy pistachios provide a climactic finish.

- ¼ cup powdered sugar or coconut sugar
- ½ teaspoon saffron threads
- ⅛ teaspoon ground cardamom
- ⅔ cup (ABOUT 12 OUNCES) plain or vanilla nondairy yogurt
- ½ teaspoon rose water (OPTIONAL)
- 4 dried figs, coarsely chopped
- 4 pitted soft dates, coarsely chopped
- ⅓ cup raw pistachios, coarsely chopped

1. Put the powdered sugar, saffron threads, and cardamom in a food processor or blender and process until the saffron is finely ground, 30 to 60 seconds.
2. Put the yogurt in a medium bowl. Add the sugar mixture and optional rose water and stir to combine.
3. Add half the figs, dates, and pistachios and stir to combine.
4. Cover and refrigerate for at least 30 minutes to let the flavors blend. Scatter the remaining figs, dates, and pistachios over the top just before serving.

Per serving: 398 calories, 11 g protein, 10 g fat (1 g sat), 73 g carbs, 73 mg sodium, 422 mg calcium, 8 g fiber

good morning muesli

makes 2 servings

This popular Swiss breakfast is a cross between porridge and granola. For this version, rolled oats are soaked in nondairy milk and yogurt in the fridge overnight (while you get to enjoy a relaxing roll in the hay). Then, in the morning, they're combined with fruit, seeds, and sweet seasonings to create a creamy breakfast cereal.

- 1 cup old-fashioned rolled oats
- 1 cup plain or vanilla nondairy milk
- ⅔ cup (ABOUT 12 OUNCES) plain or vanilla nondairy yogurt
- 2 teaspoons ground flaxseeds or flaxseed meal
- 1 large apple, coarsely chopped
- ¼ cup nuts (SUCH AS ALMONDS, PECANS, OR WALNUTS), coarsely chopped
- 2 tablespoons raisins, or 1 tablespoon dried currants
- 2 tablespoons dried cranberries or cherries
- Ground cinnamon
- Maple syrup

1. Put the oats, milk, yogurt, and flaxseeds in a medium bowl and stir to combine. Cover and refrigerate for 8 to 12 hours.
2. Stir the oat mixture. Add the apple, nuts, raisins, and cranberries and stir to combine.
3. Evenly divide the oat mixture between two bowls and top with cinnamon and maple syrup. Serve immediately.

Per serving: 404 calories, 14 g protein, 14 g fat (2 g sat), 59 g carbs, 94 mg sodium, 614 mg calcium, 9 g fiber
Note: Analysis doesn't include ground cinnamon or maple syrup to taste.

grab-bag granola

makes 4 cups, 8 servings

Store-bought granola often contains excessive amounts of sugar, salt, and oil, but when you make it yourself, you control what's in it (and who doesn't like a little control?). As the granola bakes, its alluring aroma will entice you like an erotic perfume. Enjoy it as a cold cereal with nondairy milk, or eat it by the handful as a post-nooky nosh.

2 cups old-fashioned rolled oats, rolled barley, rolled spelt, or rolled triticale
½ cup oat bran or wheat bran
½ cup sliced raw almonds
½ cup raw sunflower seeds
¼ cup ground flaxseeds or flaxseed meal
¾ teaspoon ground cinnamon
¾ teaspoon ground fenugreek
⅛ teaspoon ground nutmeg
¼ cup coconut water or apple juice
2 tablespoons maple syrup
2 tablespoons sunflower oil or other oil
½ teaspoon almond extract
½ teaspoon vanilla extract
½ cup dried fruit (SUCH AS CHERRIES, CRANBERRIES, CURRANTS, RAISINS, CHOPPED DATES OR APRICOTS, OR A COMBINATION)

1. Preheat the oven to 325 degrees F. Line a baking sheet with parchment paper or a silicone baking mat.
2. Put the rolled oats, oat bran, almonds, sunflower seeds, flaxseeds, cinnamon, fenugreek, and nutmeg in a large bowl and stir to combine.
3. Put the coconut water, maple syrup, oil, almond extract, and vanilla extract in a small bowl and whisk to combine. Pour over the oat mixture and stir until the oats are evenly moistened.
4. Transfer to the lined baking sheet and spread into a single layer with a metal spatula.
5. Bake for 20 minutes. Remove from the oven. Stir with the spatula and spread into a single layer again. Bake for 20 to 25 minutes longer, until golden brown and dry.
6. Sprinkle the dried fruit over the top and stir until evenly distributed. Let cool completely. Store in an airtight container at room temperature.

Per serving: 190 calories, 5 g protein, 10 g fat (1 g sat), 22 g carbs, 11 mg sodium, 38 mg calcium, 4 g fiber

avocado toast with coconut bacon

makes 2 servings

Sweet-and-smoky coconut bacon has been a game-changer for vegans who miss the taste of bacon, and it's surprisingly easy to make. In this recipe, the crispy morsels are used as a topping for toast that's been slathered with mashed avocado. It will rock your world!

COCONUT BACON

¾ teaspoon maple syrup
½ teaspoon reduced-sodium tamari or coconut aminos
¼ teaspoon chili powder or smoked or sweet paprika
½ cup unsweetened coconut chips

AVOCADO TOAST

1 avocado, diced
Juice of ½ lemon (ABOUT 2 TABLESPOONS)
Sea salt
Crushed red pepper flakes
2 slices whole-grain bread, toasted

1. To make the coconut bacon, preheat the oven to 325 degrees F. Line a baking sheet with parchment paper or a silicone baking mat.
2. Put the maple syrup, tamari, and chili powder in a small bowl and stir to combine. Add the coconut chips and stir until they're evenly coated.
3. Transfer to the lined baking sheet and spread into a single layer with a metal spatula. Bake for 10 to 12 minutes, stirring every 5 minutes, until the coconut chips are golden brown. Watch closely during the last 2 minutes of baking to avoid burning.
4. Remove from the oven. Let cool completely. The coconut bacon will become crispier as it cools.
5. To make the avocado toast, put the avocado and lemon juice in a small bowl and mash with a fork until it's as smooth or chunky as you like. Season with salt and red pepper flakes to taste.
6. Spread the avocado mixture evenly over the toast and top with the coconut bacon. Serve immediately.

Per serving: 325 calories, 7 g protein, 23 g fat (7 g sat), 25 g carbs, 202 mg sodium, 49 mg calcium, 10 g fiber
Note: Analysis doesn't include sea salt or crushed red pepper flakes to taste.

turn-ons When it comes to romance, coconut bacon is a bit of a player. Enjoy it as a topping for soups, salads, sandwiches, sides, and main dishes. You'll be glad you indulged.

AVOCADO TOAST WITH TOMATO: Short on time? Skip the foreplay. Ditch the coconut bacon and head right to the main event. Spread the toast with the avocado mixture and, for a beautiful finish, scatter 2 tablespoons of diced tomato over the top.

fruit-n-nut rice cakes

makes 2 servings

This combo is a little bit sweet, a little bit tart. Hey, that sounds just like you! Tangy goji berries pair up with sweet banana and luxurious nut butter for a memorable ménage à trois. A crunchy rice cake is the vehicle that drives this beauty into your eager mouth. It's ideal for a quick snack or an on-the-go breakfast when time is of the essence.

2 tablespoons nut butter (SUCH AS ALMOND, CASHEW, OR PEANUT)
2 rice cakes
1 tablespoon raw sunflower seeds
1 tablespoon dried goji berries, raisins, or cranberries
Ground cinnamon
1 banana, thinly sliced

1. Spread the nut butter evenly over each rice cake.
2. Scatter the sunflower seeds and goji berries over the top, then gently press them into the nut butter with your fingers.
3. Sprinkle with cinnamon and top with the banana. Serve immediately.

Per serving: 269 calories, 6 g protein, 11 g fat (1 g sat), 40 g carbs, 60 mg sodium, 14 mg calcium, 5 g fiber
Note: Analysis doesn't include ground cinnamon to taste.

strawberry-cashew cream cheese spread

makes 2 cups, 8 servings

Homemade cashew cream cheese is combined with juicy strawberries to create this sinfully good spread. It makes a terrific topping for toast or bagels, as well as a dip for sliced fresh fruit or celery sticks. Aw, heck, just smear it on your lover and lick it off. Yeah, it's that good!

1 cup sliced strawberries

¼ cup powdered sugar, coconut sugar, or agave nectar

1½ teaspoons vanilla extract

1 cup raw cashews, soaked in water for at least 1 hour and drained

¼ cup water or coconut water

1 tablespoon nutritional yeast flakes

1 tablespoon lemon juice

Pinch sea salt

1. Put the strawberries, powdered sugar, and vanilla extract in a small bowl and stir to combine. Let sit for 5 minutes to macerate.
2. Put the cashews, water, nutritional yeast, lemon juice, and salt in a food processor and process until smooth. Scrape down the container with a silicone spatula and process for 15 seconds longer.
3. Add the strawberry mixture and process until smooth. Transfer to an airtight container and refrigerate for at least 30 minutes before serving to let the flavors blend.

HERBED CASHEW CREAM CHEESE SPREAD: Omit the strawberries, powdered sugar, and vanilla extract. When blending the cashew mixture, add an additional 3 tablespoons of water, an additional tablespoon of nutritional yeast flakes, ½ teaspoon of onion powder, and ½ teaspoon of garlic powder. Transfer to an airtight container and stir in 2 tablespoons of chopped fresh basil or parsley and 1 thinly sliced green onion or 2 tablespoons of finely chopped chives.

Per serving: 132 calories, 3 g protein, 8 g fat (1 g sat), 11 g carbs, 36 mg sodium, 12 mg calcium, 1 g fiber

brunch in bed

Whether you prefer an early morning breakfast or a midmorning brunch, your first meal of the day is really the most important one. After all, unless you indulged after a late-night booty call, you haven't eaten for the past eight hours. The recipes in this section require a bit of foreplay, so they're best saved for leisurely mornings when there's time for a slow hand.

vanilla-almond french toast

makes 4 slices, 2 servings

You can quickly bang out the batter for this French toast by simply tossing the ingredients in a blender. If you've got maca powder handy, invite it into the mix—it will ramp up the flavor along with your libido. Serve the French toast topped with maple syrup, fresh berries, sliced fruit, or a dusting of powdered sugar. Ooh là là!

- ⅔ cup water or coconut water
- ⅓ cup whole raw almonds
- 3 pitted soft dates (PREFERABLY MEDJOOL)
- 1 tablespoon maca powder (OPTIONAL)
- 2 teaspoons vanilla extract
- 1 teaspoon ground flaxseeds or flaxseed meal
- ¼ teaspoon almond extract
- ¼ teaspoon sea salt
- 4 slices whole-grain bread

1. Put the water, almonds, dates, optional maca powder, vanilla extract, flaxseeds, almond extract, and salt in a blender and process until smooth. Scrape down the container with a silicone spatula and process for 15 seconds longer.
2. Pour into a 13 x 9-inch baking pan. Put the bread in the baking pan and flip over each slice to evenly coat both sides. Let the bread soak in the mixture for 1 minute.
3. Lightly oil a large cast-iron or nonstick skillet or griddle or mist it with cooking spray. Heat over medium heat.
4. When the skillet is hot, put in the bread and cook until golden brown on the bottom, 2 to 3 minutes. You will need to cook the bread in several batches depending on the size of the skillet. Flip the slices over with a metal spatula and cook until golden brown on the other side, 2 to 3 minutes. Serve hot.

Per serving: 207 calories, 9 g protein, 5 g fat (1 g sat), 33 g carbs, 453 mg sodium, 72 mg calcium, 6 g fiber

berry nice-and-spice pancakes

makes 4 pancakes, 2 servings

Forget going to the diner. Instead, whip up a batch of these light and fluffy pancakes for your worthy paramour. They're flavored with vanilla and spice and studded with sweet and juicy berries. And what stud or studette can resist sweet and juicy?

2 cups unbleached all-purpose flour or whole wheat pastry flour

1½ tablespoons baking powder

1 teaspoon ground cinnamon

½ teaspoon ground cardamom or ginger

Pinch sea salt

2 cups plain or vanilla nondairy milk

1 tablespoon maple syrup

1½ teaspoons vanilla extract

1 cup fresh or frozen berries (SUCH AS BLACKBERRIES, BLUEBERRIES, RASPBERRIES, SLICED STRAWBERRIES, OR MIXED BERRIES)

1. Put the flour, baking powder, cinnamon, cardamom, and salt in a large bowl and whisk to combine.
2. Add the milk, maple syrup, and vanilla extract and whisk until just combined (a few lumps are fine; don't overmix or the pancakes will be tough). Gently stir in the berries. Let the batter sit for 5 minutes.
3. Lightly oil a large cast-iron or nonstick skillet or griddle or mist it with cooking spray. Heat over medium heat.
4. When the skillet is hot, pour in the batter using ½ cup for each pancake. You will need to cook the pancakes in several batches depending on the size of the skillet. Oil the skillet again between batches. Cook until the edges of the pancakes are slightly dry and bubbles appear on top, 2 to 3 minutes. Flip the pancakes over with a metal spatula and cook until golden brown on the other side, 2 to 3 minutes. Serve hot.

turn-ons For gluten-free pancakes, replace the unbleached all-purpose flour with buckwheat flour. If you prefer to use a gluten-free flour blend, add ¾ teaspoon of xanthan gum to the dry ingredients.

Per serving: 590 calories, 15 g protein, 4 g fat (0.2 g sat), 118 g carbs, 165 mg sodium, 991 mg calcium, 9 g fiber

egg-free scramble with chiles and greens

makes 4 servings

Eggs are a symbol of fertility, but you can boost your prowess even more without them. The tofu and greens in this scrumptious scramble will give you calcium and protein for miles, and the spicy chiles will have you crowing like a proud rooster. Want to turn up the heat even more? Douse your serving with hot sauce!

1 pound extra-firm tofu
2 tablespoons nutritional yeast flakes
1 tablespoon reduced-sodium tamari or coconut aminos
½ teaspoon ground turmeric
¾ cup diced red or yellow onion
2 jalapeño chiles, cut in half lengthwise, seeded, and thinly sliced
1 tablespoon olive oil, or ¼ cup low-sodium vegetable broth
1 tablespoon minced garlic
2 cups stemmed and thinly sliced kale or mustard greens, lightly packed
¼ cup chopped fresh basil, cilantro, or parsley, lightly packed
Sea salt
Freshly ground black pepper

1. Crumble the tofu into a small bowl. Add the nutritional yeast, tamari, and turmeric and stir to combine.
2. Put the onion, chiles, oil, and garlic in a large cast-iron or nonstick skillet and cook over medium-high heat, stirring occasionally, for 2 minutes.
3. Add the tofu mixture and cook, stirring occasionally, for 5 minutes.
4. Add the kale and basil and cook, stirring occasionally, until the kale has wilted and the other vegetables are tender, 3 to 5 minutes. Season with salt and pepper to taste. Serve hot.

turn-ons If you're a fan of peppery arugula, replace the kale with 4 cups of baby arugula or coarsely chopped mature arugula, lightly packed.

Per serving: 185 calories, 16 g protein, 11 g fat (1 g sat), 11 g carbs, 203 mg sodium, 264 mg calcium, 3 g fiber
Note: Analysis doesn't include sea salt or freshly ground black pepper to taste.

rum banana roll-ups

makes 2 servings

The addition of rum in these healthy roll-ups may seem a little naughty first thing in the morning, but that's perfect for a sexy devil like you. This swoon-worthy blend of yogurt, dates, almonds, and coconut wrapped in a flour tortilla and topped with rum-soaked bananas will get you stoked for the day or your next escapade.

RUM BANANAS

2 large bananas, cut into 1-inch slices
¼ cup coconut water or water
1 tablespoon agave nectar or maple syrup
½ teaspoon ground cinnamon
2 tablespoons rum (LIGHT, DARK, OR COCONUT RUM)

ROLL-UPS

½ cup plain or vanilla nondairy yogurt
¼ cup coarsely chopped soft dates
¼ cup sliced almonds, raw or toasted
3 tablespoons unsweetened coconut chips, toasted, or 1 tablespoon unsweetened shredded dried coconut, toasted
½ teaspoon vanilla extract, or ¼ teaspoon almond extract
2 (8-INCH OR LARGER) flour tortillas

1. To make the rum bananas, put the bananas and coconut water in a large cast-iron or nonstick skillet and cook over medium heat, stirring occasionally, for 2 minutes.
2. Add the agave nectar and cinnamon, decrease the heat to low, and cook, stirring occasionally, for 2 minutes.
3. Add the rum and cook, stirring occasionally, until the bananas are soft, about 1 minute. Alternatively, flambé the banana mixture by carefully igniting it and letting the alcohol burn off before serving (see the safety tips on page 207).

4 To make the filling, put the yogurt, dates, almonds, coconut, and vanilla extract in a small bowl and stir to combine.

5 For easier rolling, warm each tortilla in a large skillet over medium heat for 1 minute per side, or microwave for 20 to 30 seconds.

6 To assemble, put each tortilla on a large plate. Spoon half the yogurt mixture in the center of each tortilla. Top with one-quarter of the rum bananas (just the bananas, not the liquid). Fold the bottom of the tortilla over the filling and continue rolling it over like a crêpe. Spoon the remaining bananas and their liquid over the top of the roll-ups. Serve immediately.

turn-ons Not in the mood for booze at breakfast? Replace the rum with an additional tablespoon of agave nectar or maple syrup. As a special treat, the rum bananas can be used as a topping for nondairy ice cream, cake, or your current love interest.

Per serving: 591 calories, 12 g protein, 19 g fat (8 g sat), 91 g carbs, 413 mg sodium, 224 mg calcium, 11 g fiber

potato latkes with applesauce

makes 4 pancakes, 2 servings

Whether you call them potato latkes or potato pancakes, you're going to love these savory patties. Most potato latkes are fried in oil, but this healthier, lighter version is oil-free and oven-baked instead. Shall we get a little fresh? Silly you, we're talking about the applesauce! But since you're slightly saucy to begin with, you can opt to omit it if you prefer.

APPLESAUCE

2 apples, peeled and diced
½ cup apple juice or water

LATKES

2 large russet potatoes, peeled
1 small yellow onion
¼ cup chopped fresh parsley, lightly packed
3 tablespoons chickpea flour, whole wheat flour, or potato starch
2 tablespoons finely chopped chives, or ¼ cup thinly sliced green onions
1½ tablespoons nutritional yeast flakes
1 teaspoon garlic powder
½ teaspoon baking powder
½ teaspoon sea salt
¼ teaspoon ground black pepper

1. To make the applesauce, put the apples and apple juice in a small saucepan and bring to a boil over medium heat. Cover, decrease the heat to low, and simmer until the apples are tender, 15 to 20 minutes. Remove from the heat, uncover, and let cool for 10 minutes.

2. Mash the apples with a potato masher or fork until they're as smooth or chunky as you like. Keep at room temperature or cover and store in the refrigerator until ready to use.

3. To make the potato latkes, preheat the oven to 425 degrees F. Line a baking sheet with parchment paper or a silicone baking mat. Fill a large bowl with cold water.

4. Finely shred the potatoes and onion using a food processor or box grater. Transfer batches to the bowl of water as you work (the cold water will prevent the potatoes from discoloring).

5 Put the potato mixture in a large colander. Using your hands, firmly squeeze the mixture to expel as much liquid as possible. (The drier the potatoes are, the crispier the latkes will be.) As you squeeze out each handful, transfer it to a medium bowl.

6 Stir the mixture with a fork to loosen it up. Add the parsley, chickpea flour, chives, nutritional yeast, garlic powder, baking powder, salt, and pepper and stir to combine.

7 Using a ¼-cup measuring cup, portion each latke by lightly filling and gently packing the mixture into the cup with the back of a spoon. Flip the measuring cup over onto the lined baking sheet and tap the cup to release the mixture. Repeat the procedure with the remaining mixture. Slightly flatten each portion with your fingers.

8 Bake on the bottom oven rack for 15 minutes. Remove from the oven and flip the latkes over with a metal spatula. Bake for 10 to 15 minutes longer, until golden brown on both sides. Serve hot, topped with the applesauce.

Per serving: 484 calories, 13 g protein, 2 g fat (0.2 g sat), 110 g carbs, 512 mg sodium, 124 mg calcium, 19 g fiber

herb-and-cheese biscuits

makes 6 biscuits

Even if you have limited baking experience, you'll find success with these tender biscuits. Infused with fragrant fresh herbs and vegan Cheddar, they're nothing short of mind-numbing bliss. Try them plain or topped with vegan butter for breakfast, or invite them to lunch or dinner. They make a welcome sidekick to soups or stews.

- ½ cup plain unsweetened nondairy milk
- 1 tablespoon cider vinegar or lemon juice
- 1¾ cups unbleached all-purpose flour or whole wheat pastry flour
- 1 tablespoon baking powder
- 1 tablespoon nutritional yeast flakes
- 1 tablespoon unbleached cane sugar
- ½ teaspoon sea salt
- 3 tablespoons vegan butter
- ⅔ cup shredded vegan Cheddar cheese
- 2 tablespoons chopped fresh parsley, or 1 tablespoon chopped fresh rosemary

1. Preheat the oven to 400 degrees F. Line a baking sheet with parchment paper or a silicone baking mat.
2. Put the milk and vinegar in a small bowl and stir to combine. Let sit for 5 minutes to thicken.
3. Put the flour, baking powder, nutritional yeast, sugar, and salt in a medium bowl and stir to combine.
4. Add the butter and work it into the flour mixture with a fork to form coarse crumbs. Add the milk mixture and stir to combine. Gently stir in the cheese and parsley.
5. Transfer to the lined baking sheet. Gently pat the dough into a 6 x 4-inch rectangle. Using a sharp knife, cut the rectangle in half widthwise, then into thirds lengthwise to yield six 2-inch squares. Keep the biscuits shaped as squares, or round the edges with your hands to make them circular.

6 Bake for 8 to 10 minutes, until the bottoms are lightly browned and the tops are firm to the touch. Serve hot, warm, or room temperature.

turn-ons For a low-fat version, decrease the amount of nondairy milk to 1/3 cup. Replace the vegan butter with 1/4 cup of plain unsweetened nondairy yogurt.

BASIL-AND-MOZZARELLA BISCUITS: Replace the parsley with 2 tablespoons of chopped fresh basil or 2 teaspoons of dried basil, and replace the Cheddar cheese with 2/3 cup of shredded vegan mozzarella cheese.

SWEET BUTTERMILK BISCUITS: Increase the amount of sugar to 2 tablespoons. Omit the parsley and cheese.

Per biscuit: 212 calories, 5 g protein, 7 g fat (2 g sat), 33 g carbs, 264 mg sodium, 154 mg calcium, 2 g fiber

seitan sausages

makes 8 sausages, 4 servings

Using vital wheat gluten instead of whole wheat flour speeds up the seitan-making process. With minimal effort, you'll have a tasty batch of vegan sausages that will have your lover clamoring for round two. Serve them for breakfast, put them on sandwiches, chop or slice them to add to soups or sauces, or crumble them over pizza, pasta, or casseroles.

- 1¼ cups vital wheat gluten
- ¼ cup chickpea flour
- 2 tablespoons nutritional yeast flakes
- 1½ teaspoons garlic powder
- 1½ teaspoons dried basil
- 1½ teaspoons dried oregano
- 1 teaspoon whole fennel seeds, or ½ teaspoon ground fennel
- ½ teaspoon crushed red pepper flakes (OPTIONAL)
- ¼ teaspoon ground black pepper
- 1 cup water or low-sodium vegetable broth
- 1 tablespoon olive oil
- 1 tablespoon reduced-sodium tamari or coconut aminos
- 1 tablespoon maple syrup
- ¼ teaspoon liquid smoke (OPTIONAL)

1. Put a collapsible steamer basket or steamer rack into a large saucepan. Add enough water to just touch the bottom of the collapsible steamer, or make the water two inches deep if using a rack. Cover the saucepan and bring to a boil over medium heat.

2. Put the vital wheat gluten, chickpea flour, nutritional yeast, garlic powder, basil, oregano, fennel seeds, optional red pepper flakes, and pepper in a large bowl and stir to combine.

3. Put the water, oil, tamari, maple syrup, and optional liquid smoke in a medium bowl and stir to combine.

4. Add the water mixture to the vital wheat gluten mixture and stir to combine. Using your hands, knead the mixture in the bowl until it forms a smooth and pliable dough, 1 to 2 minutes. Let the dough rest for 5 minutes.

5 Cut eight 6 x 6-inch pieces of parchment paper and aluminum foil. On a work surface, put a piece of parchment paper on top of each piece of aluminum foil.

6 Put ¼ cup of the sausage mixture lengthwise in the center of each parchment paper. Using your hands, shape each portion into a 4-inch log. Fold over the edges of the parchment paper around the log, then roll up the aluminum foil to enclose the log completely. Twist the ends to secure it (like a piece of wrapped candy).

7 Put the wrapped sausages in the steamer, cover, and steam for 25 minutes. Remove from the heat. Let the sausages sit in the covered saucepan for 5 minutes. Transfer to a large plate and let cool for 10 minutes. Remove and discard the sausage wrappers. Serve hot.

turn-ons The sausages are ready to eat after they've been steamed, but if you prefer, they can be cooked further in an oiled skillet over medium heat until lightly browned all over.

Per serving: 130 calories, 12 g protein, 4 g fat (1 g sat), 12 g carbs, 187 mg sodium, 40 mg calcium, 2 g fiber

tempeh bacon

makes 8 slices, 4 servings

Thin slices of tempeh are marinated in a savory blend, then oven-baked to perfection. Although you could slide this roguish bacon between the sheets, it's much better slid between two slices of bread in the missionary BLT position. But you don't have to stick to the tried and true. This bacon holds its own paired with tofu scramble or crumbled over salads, soups, or casseroles.

2 tablespoons reduced-sodium tamari or coconut aminos
1½ tablespoons cider vinegar
1 tablespoon maple syrup
1 teaspoon toasted sesame oil
1 teaspoon garlic powder
1 teaspoon chipotle chile powder or smoked or sweet paprika
¼ teaspoon ground black pepper
¼ teaspoon liquid smoke (OPTIONAL)
1 package (8 OUNCES) **tempeh**

1. To make the marinade, put the tamari, vinegar, maple syrup, oil, garlic powder, chile powder, pepper, and optional liquid smoke in an 8-inch square baking pan and whisk to combine.
2. Cut the tempeh lengthwise into eight slices. Put it in the baking pan, then flip over each slice to evenly coat both sides.
3. Put the baking pan in the refrigerator and let the tempeh marinate for at least 1 hour.
4. Preheat the oven to 400 degrees F. Line a baking sheet with parchment paper or a silicone baking mat.
5. Transfer the tempeh to the lined baking sheet. Spoon any remaining marinade over it.
6. Bake for 15 minutes. Remove from the oven and flip the tempeh over with a fork. Bake for 10 to 15 minutes longer, until golden brown and crispy around the edges. Serve hot or cold.

Per serving: 146 calories, 12 g protein, 7 g fat (1 g sat), 10 g carbs, 363 mg sodium, 79 mg calcium, 0 g fiber

banana bread

makes 8 slices

When life gives you overripe bananas, make banana bread! It's moist and delectable and will keep those good vibrations going all day long. Feeling particularly decadent? Top a slice with a scoop of nondairy ice cream and a drizzle of maple syrup. It's orgasmic!

- 1 large banana, broken into pieces
- ½ cup plain coconut milk beverage or coconut water
- 1 tablespoon sunflower oil or other oil
- 1 tablespoon cider vinegar
- 1 teaspoon vanilla extract
- 1½ cups whole wheat pastry flour
- ½ cup unbleached cane sugar or coconut sugar
- 2 teaspoons baking soda
- 1 teaspoon ground cinnamon
- ¼ teaspoon sea salt

1. Preheat the oven to 350 degrees F. Lightly oil an 8 x 4 x 2½-inch loaf pan or mist it with cooking spray.
2. Put the banana in a large bowl and coarsely mash it with a fork. Measure out ¾ cup of the mashed banana and store any extra for a snack or to use in a smoothie.
3. Put the measured banana back in the bowl. Add the milk, oil, vinegar, and vanilla extract and whisk to combine.
4. Add the flour, sugar, baking soda, cinnamon, and salt and whisk to combine.
5. Pour the batter into the prepared loaf pan and smooth the top with a silicone spatula.
6. Bake for 25 to 30 minutes, until a toothpick inserted in the center comes out clean. Let cool in the pan for 5 minutes. Loosen the sides of the loaf with a knife, then invert the pan onto a rack, letting the loaf release naturally from the pan. Serve warm or room temperature.

BLUEBERRY-BANANA BREAD: Add ½ cup of fresh or frozen blueberries (do not thaw).

Per slice: 417 calories, 9 g protein, 7 g fat (3 g sat), 78 g carbs, 376 mg sodium, 6 mg calcium, 9 g fiber

raspberry, chocolate chip, and yogurt scones

makes 8 scones

These deluxe gluten-free scones are bejeweled with whole raspberries and chocolate chips. Talk about making your heart race! Enjoy one over a cup of tea or coffee. Your sweetie won't be able to resist nibbling the crumbs from the corners of your lips.

- 3 tablespoons warm water
- 1 tablespoon ground gold flaxseeds or gold flaxseed meal
- 2¼ cups blanched almond flour
- ⅓ cup tapioca starch
- 2 tablespoons coconut flour
- 1 teaspoon baking powder
- 1 teaspoon baking soda
- ¼ teaspoon sea salt
- 1 container (6 OUNCES) plain or vanilla nondairy yogurt
- 1½ tablespoons agave nectar or maple syrup
- 1 teaspoon lemon juice or cider vinegar
- 1 teaspoon vanilla extract
- ⅓ cup fresh or frozen raspberries (DO NOT THAW)
- ⅓ cup vegan chocolate chips, or ¼ cup cacao nibs

1. Preheat the oven to 350 degrees F. Line a baking sheet with parchment paper or a silicone baking mat.
2. Put the water and flaxseeds in a small bowl and whisk to combine. Let sit for 10 minutes to thicken into a gel.
3. Put the almond flour, tapioca starch, coconut flour, baking powder, baking soda, and salt in a large bowl and stir to combine.
4. Add the flaxseed mixture, yogurt, agave nectar, lemon juice, and vanilla extract and stir to form a soft dough. Gently stir in the raspberries and chocolate chips.

5 Transfer to the lined baking sheet. Gently pat the dough into a 9-inch circle. Cut the circle into eight wedges with a sharp knife, then gently separate the wedges, spacing them two inches apart.

6 Bake for 25 to 30 minutes, until lightly browned around the edges. Let cool for 15 minutes. Serve warm or room temperature. Store leftover scones in an airtight container at room temperature or in the refrigerator.

turn-ons For a wheat-based version, replace the almond flour, tapioca starch, and coconut flour with 2½ cups of unbleached all-purpose flour or whole wheat pastry flour.

CHERRY, CHOCOLATE CHIP, AND YOGURT SCONES: Replace the raspberries with ½ cup of pitted fresh or frozen cherries (do not thaw).

Per scone: 160 calories, 4 g protein, 7 g fat (2 g sat), 20 g carbs, 229 mg sodium, 88 mg calcium, 3 g fiber

cappuccino-chip muffins

makes 6 muffins

Make an extra cup of coffee in the morning and save it to make these enchanting muffins. If "warm, dark, and succulent" describes your cuppa, you've met your match.

- 3 tablespoons warm water
- 1 teaspoon chia seeds
- 1 cup unbleached all-purpose flour or whole wheat pastry flour
- 2½ tablespoons unbleached cane sugar
- 1 tablespoon cacao powder or unsweetened cocoa powder
- 1¼ teaspoons baking powder
- ¼ teaspoon ground cinnamon
- ¼ teaspoon sea salt
- ½ cup cold coffee
- 1½ tablespoons sunflower oil or other oil
- ½ teaspoon vanilla extract
- ½ cup vegan chocolate chips, or ⅓ cup cacao nibs

1. Preheat the oven to 400 degrees F. Line a standard six-cup muffin tin with paper or silicone liners, or lightly oil it or mist it with cooking spray.
2. Put the water and chia seeds in a small bowl and stir to combine. Let sit for 10 minutes to thicken into a gel.
3. Put the flour, 2 tablespoons of the sugar, and the cacao powder, baking powder, cinnamon, and salt in a medium bowl and whisk to combine.
4. Add the chia seed mixture, coffee, oil, and vanilla extract and whisk to combine. Gently stir in the chocolate chips.
5. Fill the prepared muffin cups three-quarters full. Sprinkle the remaining 1½ teaspoons of sugar over the tops of the muffins. Bake for 18 to 20 minutes, until a toothpick inserted in the center of a muffin comes out clean. Let cool in the pan for 5 minutes, then transfer to a rack. Serve warm or room temperature. Store leftover muffins in an airtight container at room temperature or in the refrigerator.

Per muffin: 297 calories, 4 g protein, 19 g fat (4 g sat), 31 g carbs, 92 mg sodium, 143 mg calcium, 2 g fiber

carrot cake muffins

makes 6 muffins

Here are some top-of-the-line stud muffins. Moist and tender, chewy and crunchy, these switch-hitters are as comfortable at the breakfast table as they are on the dessert cart. If you're feeling demure, serve them plain. But if you want to get a wee bit wild, plop some nondairy yogurt or Whipped Coconut Cream (page 215) on top.

2 tablespoons warm water
2 teaspoons ground flaxseeds or flaxseed meal
1½ cups blanched almond flour
3 tablespoons arrowroot starch
1½ teaspoons baking powder
1 teaspoon ground cinnamon
½ teaspoon ground ginger
¼ teaspoon ground cloves
¼ teaspoon ground nutmeg
¼ teaspoon sea salt
2½ tablespoons plain nondairy milk
2½ tablespoons maple syrup
1 teaspoon vanilla extract
¾ cup coarsely grated carrots, lightly packed
¼ cup coarsely chopped raw walnuts
2 tablespoon raisins

1. Preheat the oven to 375 degrees F. Line a standard six-cup muffin tin with paper or silicone liners, or lightly oil it or mist it with cooking spray.
2. Put the water and flaxseeds in a small bowl and whisk to combine. Let sit for 10 minutes to thicken into a gel.
3. Put the almond flour, arrowroot starch, baking powder, cinnamon, ginger, cloves, nutmeg, and salt in a large bowl and whisk to combine.
4. Add the flaxseed mixture, milk, maple syrup, and vanilla extract and whisk to combine. Gently stir in the carrots, walnuts, and raisins.
5. Fill the prepared muffin cups three-quarters full. Bake for 22 to 25 minutes, until a toothpick inserted in the center of a muffin comes out clean. Let cool in the pan for 5 minutes, then transfer to a rack. Serve warm or room temperature. Store leftover muffins in an airtight container at room temperature or in the refrigerator.

Per muffin: 145 calories, 2 g protein, 8 g fat (2 g sat), 16 g carbs, 98 mg sodium, 72 mg calcium, 3 g fiber

afternoon delights

Dig a romantic rendezvous in the morning, afternoon, evening, or night? Then you'll need to refuel by midday to stay at the top of your game. The soups, salads, and sandwiches in this section will satisfy your lunchtime desires so you can perform at your peak any time you like.

greek chickpea salad

makes 2 servings

Greek salad is traditionally garnished with crumbled feta cheese, but this veganized version calls for protein-packed chickpeas instead. According to the Greeks, legumes boost libido. If you want to look like a Greek god or goddess or simply feel like one, dig in!

1 can (15 OUNCES) chickpeas, drained and rinsed
1 cucumber, cut lengthwise into quarters and thickly sliced
1 cup halved cherry tomatoes, or 1 cup diced tomatoes
½ cup diced red onion
⅓ cup pitted kalamata or black olives, halved lengthwise
¼ cup chopped fresh mint or parsley leaves, lightly packed
Zest and juice of 1 lemon (ABOUT 1 TABLESPOON ZEST AND ¼ CUP JUICE)
1 tablespoon olive oil
1 tablespoon minced garlic
1 teaspoon dried oregano
Sea salt
Freshly ground black pepper

1. Put the chickpeas, cucumber, tomatoes, onion, olives, and mint in a large bowl and stir to combine.
2. Add the lemon zest and juice, oil, garlic, and oregano and stir to combine. Season with salt and pepper to taste. Serve immediately.

FATTOUSH: Lightly toast 1 (6-inch) pita bread, then tear it into bite-sized pieces. Add to the salad just before serving (so the bread doesn't get soggy) and gently stir to combine.

Per serving: 434 calories, 18 g protein, 14 g fat (2 g sat), 63 g carbs, 221 mg sodium, 175 mg calcium, 17 g fiber
Note: Analysis doesn't include sea salt or freshly ground black pepper to taste.

avocado, fennel, and citrus salad

makes 2 servings

For this simple and refreshing salad, thinly sliced fennel is briefly marinated in a tangy vinaigrette to soften its texture and mellow its flavor. Then it's caressed by juicy citrus segments, avocado, and mint leaves for an orgy of tastes and textures.

1 large orange or red grapefruit
1½ teaspoons olive oil
½ teaspoon whole-grain mustard or Dijon mustard
Sea salt
Freshly ground black pepper
1 fennel bulb
1 avocado, thinly sliced
2 tablespoons mint leaves

1. If using an orange, zest it over a large bowl. If using a grapefruit, don't remove the zest. Cut the fruit into segments over the bowl to catch the juices, then cut each segment in half and set aside.
2. Add the olive oil and mustard to the orange zest and juice and whisk to combine. Season with salt and pepper to taste and set aside.
3. To prepare the fennel, slice off the fronds and coarsely chop them. Set aside.
4. Cut the fennel bulb into quarters lengthwise, then remove and discard the core. Thinly slice each quarter and add to the orange juice mixture. Gently toss to coat the fennel. Let sit for 10 minutes to marinate.
5. Add the reserved fennel fronds and citrus segments, avocado, and mint leaves and gently toss to combine. Serve immediately.

turn-ons For a heartier salad, serve the fennel mixture over 3 cups of baby arugula or baby mixed greens, lightly packed.

Per serving: 321 calories, 5 g protein, 23 g fat (5 g sat), 29 g carbs, 69 mg sodium, 122 mg calcium, 13 g fiber
Note: Analysis doesn't include sea salt or freshly ground black pepper to taste.

aphrodite salad with pomegranate dressing

makes 2 servings

Aphrodite, the Greek goddess of love, beauty, and pleasure, is credited with planting the first pomegranate tree. She no doubt would have approved of this stunning salad, which arouses all the senses. Tender baby greens are tossed with fresh berries, dried fruits, and crunchy nuts, then drizzled with a seductive pomegranate dressing.

POMEGRANATE DRESSING

¼ cup pomegranate seeds

1½ tablespoons olive oil or walnut oil

1 tablespoon cider vinegar

1 tablespoon agave nectar, maple syrup, or coconut sugar

1 tablespoon finely diced shallot or red or yellow onion

SALAD

3 cups mixed baby greens, lightly packed

1 cup fresh berries (SUCH AS BLUEBERRIES, BLACKBERRIES, RASPBERRIES, OR SLICED STRAWBERRIES)

½ cup thinly sliced celery

¼ cup coarsely chopped dried fruit (SUCH AS CHERRIES, CRANBERRIES, DATES, OR FIGS)

¼ cup pomegranate seeds

¼ cup alfalfa sprouts

¼ cup sliced almonds or coarsely chopped walnuts

1. To make the dressing, put all the ingredients in a blender and process until smooth. Scrape down the container with a silicone spatula and process for 15 seconds longer.

2. To make the salad, put the greens, berries, celery, dried fruit, and pomegranate seeds in a large bowl and gently toss to combine. Scatter the alfalfa sprouts and almonds over the top. Drizzle with the dressing and serve immediately.

Per serving: 340 calories, 7 g protein, 20 g fat (2 g sat), 38 g carbs, 42 mg sodium, 44 mg calcium, 6 g fiber

cleopatra salad with hemp seed dressing

makes 2 servings

Cleopatra is well known for her love affairs with Julius Caesar and Marcus Antonius. These tumultuous relationships provided the inspiration for this novel twist on the classic tossed Caesar salad.

CREAMY HEMP SEED DRESSING

3 tablespoons water
2 tablespoons lemon juice
1½ tablespoons hemp seeds
1 tablespoon raw pine nuts
½ teaspoon Dijon mustard
1 large clove garlic, coarsely chopped
¼ teaspoon dried basil
Pinch sea salt
Pinch ground black pepper

SALAD

4 cups thinly sliced romaine lettuce, lightly packed
1½ teaspoons nutritional yeast flakes
½ cup shredded beets, lightly packed
½ cup shredded carrots, lightly packed
½ cup shredded red cabbage, lightly packed
½ cup diced zucchini
¼ cup pine nuts, toasted
¼ cup coarsely chopped dried figs

1. To make the dressing, put all the ingredients in a blender and process until smooth. Scrape down the container with a silicone spatula and process for 15 seconds longer.
2. To make the salad, put the lettuce in a large bowl and sprinkle the nutritional yeast over the top. Drizzle the dressing over the mixture and gently toss to combine.
3. Add the beets, carrots, red cabbage, and zucchini and gently toss to combine. Scatter the pine nuts and figs over the top and serve immediately.

Per serving: 664 calories, 21 g protein, 41 g fat (2 g sat), 65 g carbs, 399 mg sodium, 160 mg calcium, 14 g fiber

pacific northwest kale salad

makes 2 servings

The Pacific Northwest states of Washington and Oregon are famous for their apples, pears, and hazelnuts. The crisp, crunchy texture of these highly prized crops is showcased in this scantily clad salad, cloaked in a sheer but provocative vinaigrette.

CIDER-AND-MUSTARD VINAIGRETTE

1 tablespoon apple cider or apple juice

1 tablespoon cider vinegar

2 teaspoons olive oil or hazelnut oil

2 teaspoons whole-grain mustard, or 1 teaspoon stone-ground mustard and ½ teaspoon mustard seeds

1 teaspoon chia seeds

½ teaspoon agave nectar

SALAD

1 apple, diced

1 pear, diced

1 teaspoon lemon juice

10 kale leaves (ANY VARIETY), stemmed and cut into thin strips

⅓ cup hazelnuts, toasted and coarsely chopped

¼ cup dried cranberries or raisins, or 2 tablespoons dried currants

1. To make the dressing, put all the ingredients in a small bowl and whisk to combine. Let sit for 10 minutes to thicken. Whisk the dressing again to break up any clumps of chia seeds.
2. Put the apple and pear in a small bowl, drizzle the lemon juice over the top, and gently toss to evenly coat.
3. To make the salad, put the kale in a large bowl. Drizzle the dressing over the kale. Using your hands, vigorously massage the kale until it begins to wilt, 3 to 5 minutes
4. Add the apple-pear mixture, hazelnuts, and cranberries and gently toss to combine. Serve immediately.

Per serving: 375 calories, 8 g protein, 14 g fat (1 g sat), 61 g carbs, 66 mg sodium, 253 mg calcium, 11 g fiber

gingery carrot soup

makes 4 servings

Carrots are an excellent source of beta-carotene, as well as vitamins C and E, zinc, and selenium. Equally significant, they impart a healthy glow that can enhance your natural sex appeal. But why keep that to yourself? This energizing, easy-to-digest soup is packed with flavorful, fragrant spices, making it a delectable choice for a lunch date.

1 pound carrots, sliced
4 cups water or low-sodium vegetable broth
1 cup diced yellow onion, or 2 medium shallots, diced
Zest and juice of 1 large orange (ABOUT 3 TABLESPOONS ZEST AND ½ CUP JUICE)
2 tablespoons peeled and grated fresh ginger
¼ teaspoon ground cinnamon
¼ teaspoon ground cardamom
1½ tablespoons nutritional yeast flakes
Sea salt

1 Put the carrots, water, onion, orange zest and juice, ginger, cinnamon, and cardamom in a large soup pot and stir to combine. Bring to a boil over high heat. Cover, decrease the heat to low, and simmer until the carrots are tender, 15 to 20 minutes.

2 Remove from the heat. Let cool for 10 minutes. Transfer half the soup to a large bowl and set aside. Put the remaining soup in a blender. Add the nutritional yeast and process until smooth. Scrape down the container with a silicone spatula and process for 15 seconds longer. Pour into the soup pot.

3 Transfer the remaining soup to the blender and process until smooth. Scrape down the container with a silicone spatula and process for 15 seconds longer. Pour into the soup pot. Season with salt to taste. Serve hot.

CURRY CARROT SOUP: Prefer spicy over sweet? Replace the cinnamon and cardamom with ½ teaspoon of curry powder.

Per serving: 121 calories, 8 g protein, 1 g fat (0.1 g sat), 24 g carbs, 88 mg sodium, 57 mg calcium, 7 g fiber
Note: Analysis doesn't include sea salt to taste.

mexican tortilla soup

makes 4 servings

Turn the heat up a notch with a bowl of this colorful soup. The smoky, tomato-based broth is loaded with beans, corn, jalapeño chile, green onions, and cilantro. Each serving is topped with crushed tortilla chips, luscious avocado, and a gentle squeeze of fresh lime juice. Are you weak in the knees yet?

1½ cups low-sodium vegetable broth
½ cup diced red onion
½ cup thinly sliced green onions
1 jalapeño chile, cut in half lengthwise, seeded, and finely diced
1 tablespoon minced garlic
1 can (28 OUNCES) **crushed tomatoes** (FOR A SMOKY FLAVOR, USE FIRE-ROASTED TOMATOES)
1 can (15 OUNCES) **beans** (SUCH AS BLACK, KIDNEY, OR PINTO)**, drained and rinsed**
⅔ cup frozen corn kernels
1½ teaspoons chili powder
1 teaspoon ground cumin
1 teaspoon dried oregano
¼ teaspoon chipotle chile powder or cayenne
½ cup chopped fresh cilantro, lightly packed
Sea salt
Freshly ground black pepper
1 cup coarsely crushed tortilla chips
1 avocado, diced
1 lime, cut into four wedges

1. Put ½ cup of the broth and the red onion, green onions, chile, and garlic in a large soup pot. Cook over medium-high heat, stirring occasionally, until the vegetables are softened, about 5 minutes.

2. Add the remaining cup of broth and the tomatoes, beans, corn, chili powder, cumin, oregano, and chipotle chile powder and stir to combine. Bring to a boil over high heat. Cover, decrease the heat to low, and simmer until the vegetables are tender, about 15 minutes.

3. Stir in the cilantro. Season with salt and pepper to taste. Serve hot, garnished with the tortilla chips, avocado, and lime.

Per serving: 383 calories, 12 g protein, 18 g fat (3 g sat), 48 g carbs, 373 mg sodium, 131 mg calcium, 13 g fiber
Note: Analysis doesn't include sea salt or freshly ground black pepper to taste.

mood-enhancing mushroom soup

makes 4 servings

Ready to get in the mood? This soup incorporates a number of vegan aphrodisiacs, including mushrooms, celery, onion, garlic, herbs, and maca. But it's the decadent flourish of creamy cashews and white wine that transforms it from healthy to nearly hedonistic.

8 ounces mushrooms, halved and thinly sliced (ABOUT 3 CUPS)
3 cups low-sodium vegetable broth
¾ cup diced celery
¾ cup diced yellow onion
2 tablespoons minced garlic
1 teaspoon dried basil or oregano
1 teaspoon dried thyme
¾ cup raw cashews, soaked in water for at least 1 hour and drained
¼ cup white wine or dry sherry (OPTIONAL)
2 tablespoons maca powder
1½ tablespoons nutritional yeast flakes
¼ cup chopped fresh parsley, lightly packed
Sea salt
Freshly ground black pepper

1. Put the mushrooms, ½ cup of the broth, and the celery, onion, garlic, basil, and thyme in a large soup pot. Cook over medium-high heat, stirring occasionally, until the vegetables are softened, about 5 minutes.
2. Add the remaining 2½ cups of broth and bring to a boil over high heat. Cover, decrease the heat to low, and simmer until the mushrooms are tender, about 20 minutes.
3. Transfer 1 cup of the hot soup to a blender. Add the cashews, optional wine, maca powder, and nutritional yeast and process until smooth. Pour into the soup pot.
4. Add the parsley and stir to combine. Simmer for 2 minutes. Season with salt and pepper to taste. Serve hot.

Per serving: 250 calories, 15 g protein, 13 g fat (3 g sat), 23 g carbs, 87 mg sodium, 63 mg calcium, 6 g fiber
Note: Analysis doesn't include sea salt or freshly ground black pepper to taste.

white bean chili

makes 4 servings

Chili doesn't have to be red and doesn't have to be made with tomatoes. If you like bucking the norm, this hearty bowl of white, not red, should be just your style. Serve it with tortilla chips, crackers, or cornbread, or maybe try all three if you lean toward the kinky side.

- 1 cup diced red or yellow onion
- 1 orange or yellow bell pepper, diced
- 1 tablespoon olive oil, or ¼ cup water
- 1 tablespoon minced garlic
- 1 teaspoon ground cumin
- 1 teaspoon dried oregano
- ½ teaspoon ground coriander
- 2 cans (15 OUNCES) white beans (SUCH AS GREAT NORTHERN OR NAVY BEANS), drained and rinsed
- 3 cups low-sodium vegetable broth
- 1 cup frozen corn kernels
- 1 can (4 OUNCES) green chiles
- ¼ cup chopped fresh cilantro, lightly packed
- 1½ tablespoons nutritional yeast flakes
- Sea salt
- Freshly ground black pepper

1. Put the onion, bell pepper, and oil in a large soup pot. Cook over medium heat, stirring occasionally, until the vegetables are softened, about 5 minutes. Add the garlic, cumin, oregano, and coriander and cook, stirring occasionally, for 1 minute.
2. Put half the beans and 1 cup of the broth in a food processor and process until smooth.
3. Add the blended mixture, remaining beans, remaining 2 cups of broth, and the corn and chiles to the soup pot and stir to combine. Cover, decrease the heat to low, and simmer until the vegetables are tender, about 20 minutes.
4. Stir in the cilantro and nutritional yeast. Season with salt and pepper to taste. Serve hot.

Per serving: 356 calories, 20 g protein, 6 g fat (1 g sat), 61 g carbs, 482 mg sodium, 138 mg calcium, 21 g fiber
Note: Analysis doesn't include sea salt or freshly ground black pepper to taste.

pho you noodle bowls

makes 4 servings

This is a veganized version of Vietnamese pho—a savory broth enhanced with tofu, leafy greens, chiles, noodles, fresh herbs, and lime juice. It's slightly salty, spicy, and citrusy. (The soup, you dirty devil, not your paramour!)

- 4 cups low-sodium vegetable broth
- 1 baby bok choy, cut into thin strips, or 2 cups baby spinach, lightly packed
- 1 cup pea pods, cut in half diagonally
- 1 package (6 OUNCES) smoked or baked tofu, cut into bite-sized cubes, or 1 cup cubed firm tofu
- 1 jalapeño chile or other chile, cut in half lengthwise and thinly sliced
- 2 tablespoons reduced-sodium tamari or coconut aminos
- 1 tablespoon rice vinegar
- 1 tablespoon peeled and grated fresh ginger
- 1 teaspoon coconut sugar or light brown sugar
- 4 ounces rice noodles, buckwheat soba noodles, or other noodles, broken in half
- 1 cup mung bean sprouts
- ¼ cup chopped fresh cilantro or mint, lightly packed
- ¼ cup roasted peanuts, coarsely chopped
- 1 lime, cut into four wedges

1. Put the broth, bok choy, pea pods, tofu, chile, tamari, vinegar, ginger, and sugar in a large soup pot and stir to combine. Bring to a boil over high heat. Decrease the heat to low and simmer, stirring occasionally, for 5 minutes.
2. Add the noodles and simmer until tender, 2 to 10 minutes (depending on the type of noodle used).
3. Stir in the sprouts and cilantro. Serve hot, garnished with the peanuts and lime wedges.

Per serving: 170 calories, 12 g protein, 7 g fat (1 g sat), 17 g carbs, 452 mg sodium, 159 mg calcium, 3 g fiber

avocado dream spread

makes 4 servings

Have an avocado fetish? Join the crowd! This pale-green spread will satisfy your wildest fantasies. It's rich, creamy, and chock-full of sun-dried tomatoes, red onion, and bell pepper. Serve generous scoops on a king-sized bed of mixed greens or baby spinach, or smear it over your favorite bread or crackers du jour.

- ⅓ cup hot water
- 5 whole sun-dried tomatoes, or ⅓ cup chopped sun-dried tomatoes (NOT PACKED IN OIL)
- 8 ounces firm or extra-firm tofu
- 1 avocado, diced
- 3 tablespoons plain unsweetened nondairy yogurt or vegan mayonnaise
- 1 tablespoon chopped fresh dill, or 1 teaspoon dried dill weed
- 1 tablespoon nutritional yeast flakes
- 1 tablespoon lemon juice
- 1½ teaspoons reduced-sodium tamari or coconut aminos
- 1 teaspoon garlic powder
- ¼ teaspoon ground black pepper
- ⅓ cup finely diced red onion
- ⅓ cup finely diced orange or red bell pepper

1. Put the water and sun-dried tomatoes in a small bowl. Let sit for 10 minutes to rehydrate and soften the tomatoes. Drain. If using whole sun-dried tomatoes, coarsely chop them and set aside.
2. Crumble the tofu into a medium bowl. Add the avocado. Using a potato masher or fork, mash the tofu and avocado until well combined but still a bit chunky.
3. Add the yogurt, dill, nutritional yeast, lemon juice, tamari, garlic powder, and pepper and stir to combine. Add the reserved sun-dried tomatoes, onion, and bell pepper and stir to combine. Store in an airtight container in the refrigerator.

Per serving: 193 calories, 9 g protein, 13 g fat (3 g sat), 12 g carbs, 153 mg sodium, 152 mg calcium, 5 g fiber

chocolate nut butter and banana paninis

makes 2 sandwiches, 2 servings

If you want to improve your sex life, give yourself the treat of chocolate, as with these extravagant paninis. Heck, just saying the name "panini" is provocative! The rush of endorphins produced by eating dark chocolate is similar to the pleasurable feelings associated with sex. So in essence, eating these paninis is a love affair!

- **¼ cup nut butter** (SUCH AS ALMOND, CASHEW, HAZELNUT, OR PEANUT)
- **1½ tablespoons cacao powder or unsweetened cocoa powder**
- **1 tablespoon maple syrup or agave nectar**
- **½ teaspoon vanilla extract**
- **4 slices whole-grain bread**
- **1 banana, thinly sliced**
- **4 teaspoons vegan butter, softened, or coconut oil, melted**

1. To make the chocolate nut butter, put the nut butter, cacao powder, maple syrup, and vanilla extract in a small bowl and stir to combine.
2. To assemble the paninis, spread the chocolate nut butter evenly over each slice of bread. Arrange the the banana on two of the slices, then top with the remaining bread, spread-side in.
3. Preheat a panini maker on medium-high heat. Alternatively, use a large cast-iron or nonstick skillet and place over medium-high heat.
4. To cook the paninis, spread half the butter over the top of the sandwiches. Put the sandwiches butter-side down in the panini maker or skillet and spread the remaining butter over the top. Close the panini maker and cook until the bread is golden brown, 3 to 5 minutes, or cook the sandwiches in the skillet for 3 minutes per side. Cut each panini in half on a diagonal. Serve hot.

turn-ons Replace the banana with ⅓ cup raspberries or sliced strawberries.

Per serving: 306 calories, 9 g protein, 11 g fat (3 g sat), 45 g carbs, 299 mg sodium, 69 mg calcium, 8 g fiber

black bean and mango lettuce wraps

makes 4 servings

Black beans, mango, bell pepper, and red onion unite in this slightly sweet, slightly spicy mixture that's wrapped in large lettuce leaves. Prefer a little nudity? Turn the lights down low, light a few candles, and serve this eye-catching salad sans the wrap on top of burritos, salads, or grains, or use it as a chunky dip for tortilla chips.

1 can (15 OUNCES) **black beans, drained and rinsed**
1 mango, peeled, pitted, and diced
¾ cup diced red bell pepper
½ cup diced red onion
¼ cup chopped fresh cilantro, lightly packed
1 jalapeño chile, seeded and finely diced
1 tablespoon minced garlic
Juice of 1 lime (ABOUT 2 TABLESPOONS)
Sea salt
Freshly ground black pepper
4 large Boston or Bibb lettuce leaves or other lettuce leaves

1. To make the salad, put the beans, mango, bell pepper, onion, cilantro, chile, garlic, and lime juice in a medium bowl and stir to combine. Season with salt and pepper to taste.

2. To assemble, put a lettuce leaf on a large plate, stem-side up. Spoon one-quarter of the salad in the center of the leaf and fold the lettuce around the salad to enclose it. Repeat with the remaining lettuce leaves and salad. Serve immediately.

Per serving: 342 calories, 16 g protein, 2 g fat (1 g sat), 71 g carbs, 9 mg sodium, 82 mg calcium, 17 g fiber
Note: Analysis doesn't include sea salt or freshly ground black pepper to taste.

italian grinders

makes 2 servings

No, we're not talking about grinding a savory Italian (although that sounds enticing). Depending on the region, these mammoth sandwiches go by various monikers, including hoagies, submarines, torpedoes, and heroes. No matter which name you prefer, you'll definitely call this veg-centric version phenomenal.

2 (6-INCH) **Italian hoagie rolls, split, or 4 slices whole-grain bread**
2 large lettuce leaves (SUCH AS ROMAINE OR LOOSELEAF)
½ cup thinly sliced orange or red bell pepper
¼ cup thinly sliced red or yellow onion
Olive oil
Red wine vinegar or balsamic vinegar
Dried basil
Dried oregano
Sea salt
Freshly ground black pepper
Sliced pickles or sliced hot peppers (SUCH AS PEPPERONCINI)
8 slices tomato
4 slices vegan mozzarella or other vegan cheese

1. Put the rolls cut-side up on a cutting board. Layer the lettuce, bell pepper, and onion on the bottom half of each roll.
2. Drizzle a little oil and vinegar over the vegetables. Sprinkle with basil, oregano, salt, and pepper as desired.
3. Add pickles as desired, then layer the tomato and cheese on top. Cover with the top half of the roll and carefully cut in half. Serve immediately.

turn-ons Enjoy your grinders on the go! Wrap them in your arms or, for less mess, with plastic wrap. Alternatively, put them in an airtight container and store in the refrigerator.

Per serving: 388 calories, 11 g protein, 13 g fat (5 g sat), 60 g carbs, 665 mg sodium, 72 mg calcium, 4 g fiber
Note: Analysis doesn't include olive oil, vinegar, basil, oregano, sea salt, freshly ground black pepper, or pickles to taste.

baked falafel sandwiches with cucumber tzatziki

makes 4 sandwiches, 4 servings

Although fried foods may seem appealing, they can deplete energy and make a person feel heavy, sluggish, and not very sexy. That's not a problem with these oven-baked falafels. Topped with creamy cucumber tzatziki sauce, these little powerballs will crank up your engines and appease all your appetites.

BAKED FALAFEL

½ small yellow onion

4 large cloves garlic

¼ cup fresh parsley or cilantro leaves or a combination, lightly packed

Zest and juice of ½ lemon (ABOUT 1½ TEASPOONS ZEST AND 2 TABLESPOONS JUICE)

1 teaspoon ground cumin

1 teaspoon ground coriander

½ teaspoon sea salt

¼ teaspoon ground black pepper

1 can (15 OUNCES) chickpeas, drained and rinsed

¼ cup chickpea flour or whole wheat flour

1 teaspoon baking powder

CUCUMBER TZATZIKI

1 container (6 OUNCES) plain unsweetened nondairy yogurt

¼ cup finely diced cucumber

1 tablespoon chopped fresh mint or dill

Sea salt

Freshly ground black pepper

SANDWICH FIXIN'S

4 pita breads

4 large lettuce leaves (SUCH AS ROMAINE OR LOOSELEAF)

1 large tomato, diced

1. Preheat the oven to 400 degrees F. Line a baking sheet with parchment paper or a silicone baking mat.

2. To make the falafel, put the onion, garlic, parsley, lemon zest and juice, cumin, coriander, salt, and pepper in a food processor and process until finely chopped. Scrape down the container with a silicone spatula. Add the chickpeas, chickpea flour, and baking powder and process until the mixture is coarsely chopped (do not purée). Cover and refrigerate for 30 minutes to let the mixture firm up slightly.

3 Portion the falafel onto the prepared baking sheet two inches apart using a heaping tablespoonful for each one (the mixture should make twelve falafel). Leave the falafel ball-shaped or slightly flatten each ball with your fingers.

4 Bake for 15 minutes. Remove from the oven and flip the falafel over with a metal spatula. Bake for 10 to 12 minutes longer, until golden brown on both sides.

5 While the falafel are baking, make the cucumber tzatziki. Put the yogurt, cucumber, and mint in a small bowl and stir to combine. Season with salt and pepper to taste.

6 To assemble each sandwich, put a lettuce leaf in the center of each pita bread. Evenly divide the falafel among them. Top with the cucumber tzatziki and tomato.

7 Serve immediately. To eat, fold the pita bread like a taco.

turn-ons To pack the sandwiches for lunch or save for a midnight snack, wrap them with plastic wrap or put them in an airtight container and store in the refrigerator.

Per serving: 361 calories, 16 g protein, 4 g fat (1 g sat), 66 g carbs, 576 mg sodium, 263 mg calcium, 9 g fiber
Note: Analysis doesn't include sea salt or freshly ground black pepper to taste.

quarter-pounder beet burgers

makes 4 burgers

Red is associated with passion, and these crimson burgers are sure to ignite yours. But they offer more than fab flavor and a rosy color. Beets contain boron and tryptophan that boost the body's sex hormones, making you feel both relaxed and aroused. Serve these plump beauties on soft, voluptuous buns (squeeze them gently), decked out with your favorite condiments.

1¼ cups water

1 cup shredded beets, lightly packed

½ cup quinoa or millet, rinsed

½ cup finely diced red or yellow onion

4 large cloves garlic, minced

1½ teaspoons Italian seasoning, or ½ teaspoon each dried basil, oregano, and rosemary

¾ teaspoon ground cumin

½ teaspoon chili powder, or ½ teaspoon smoked or sweet paprika

1½ tablespoons ground flaxseeds or flaxseed meal

½ cup coarsely ground walnuts

1½ tablespoons nutritional yeast flakes

Sea salt

Freshly ground black pepper

1. Put 1 cup of the water and the beets, quinoa, onion, garlic, Italian seasoning, cumin, and chili powder in a large saucepan and stir to combine. Bring to a boil over high heat. Cover, decrease the heat to low, and cook until the quinoa is tender and all the water is absorbed, 20 to 25 minutes. Remove from the heat, uncover the saucepan, and let cool for 10 minutes.

2. Put the remaining ¼ cup of water and the flaxseeds in a small bowl and stir to combine. Let sit for 10 minutes to thicken into a gel.

3. Transfer the beet mixture to a large bowl. Add the flaxseed mixture, walnuts, and nutritional yeast. Using a spoon or fork, stir to combine, slightly mashing the mixture against the side of the bowl to help bind it together. Season with salt and pepper to taste.

4 Line a baking sheet with parchment paper or a silicone baking mat.

5 Using a ½-cup measuring cup, portion each patty by lightly filling the cup with the burger mixture and gently packing it with the back of a spoon. Flip the measuring cup over onto the lined baking sheet and tap the cup to release the burger mixture. Lightly flatten each portion into a patty. Refrigerate for at least 1 hour to let the patties firm up slightly.

6 Preheat the oven to 400 degrees F.

7 Bake the burgers for 15 minutes. Remove from the oven and flip the burgers over with a metal spatula. Bake for 15 to 20 minutes longer, until golden brown on both sides.

BEET SLIDERS: There's nothing quite like a good slider, is there? Use a ¼-cup measuring cup to portion each patty (there will be eight patties in all). Bake for 10 minutes, flip the patties over, and bake for 10 to 12 minutes longer, until golden brown on both sides.

Per burger: 304 calories, 15 g protein, 15 g fat (2 g sat), 31 g carbs, 49 mg sodium, 49 mg calcium, 10 g fiber
Note: Analysis doesn't include sea salt or freshly ground black pepper to taste.

naughty nibbles

Although eating between meals is often maligned, many nutrition experts believe it's better for our metabolism if we graze throughout the day rather than stuff down three large feasts. These nibbles are perfect for that. They're also great for a little something-something to whet your appetite before the main dish or to quell any hunger pangs after an amorous encounter. Nibble your sweetie pie's ear or one of these snacks—your choice!

sweet-and-savory snack mix

makes 8 servings

If you're not sure whether you want to nibble something sweet or something savory, don't worry—this quick mix combines both. Problem solved! When it comes to choosing sweet or savory lovers, however, you're on your own.

- **1 recipe Coconut Bacon** (PAGE 102)
- **½ cup banana chips**
- **½ cup roasted peanuts**
- **½ cup vegan chocolate chips**

1. Prepare the coconut bacon according to the recipe. Let cool completely, then transfer to a medium bowl.
2. Add the remaining ingredients and stir to combine. Store in an airtight container at room temperature.

Per serving: 89 calories, 3 g protein, 6 g fat (2 g sat), 7 g carbs, 20 mg sodium, 10 mg calcium, 2 g fiber

apricot delights

makes 12 balls, 4 servings

Turkish delight is a chewy candy traditionally made with chopped dates and nuts and coated with a powdery starch. They were the inspiration for these wholesome, finger-sized treats, which are made with dried fruits, pistachios, hemp seeds, coconut, and mandarin orange. Here's one guilty pleasure you don't need to feel guilty about!

- 1 medium mandarin or satsuma orange
- 3 tablespoons whole raw almonds
- 1½ tablespoons unsweetened shredded dried coconut
- ½ cup raw pistachios
- 2 tablespoons hemp seeds
- ¾ cup dried apricots
- ½ cup pitted soft dates
- ¾ teaspoon ground cinnamon

1. Zest the orange and set the zest aside. Juice the orange, measure out 4 teaspoons of juice, and set aside. (Drink the remaining juice or store it in the refrigerator to enjoy another time.)
2. Put the almonds in a food processor and process until coarsely chopped. Scrape down the container with a silicone spatula. Add the reserved orange zest and coconut and process until finely chopped, about 1 minute. Transfer to a small plate and set aside.
3. Put the pistachios in the food processor and process until coarsely chopped. Transfer to a medium bowl. Stir in the hemp seeds.
4. Put the apricots, dates, reserved orange juice, and cinnamon in the food processor and process until the mixture comes together to form a ball, 1 to 2 minutes.
5. Add the apricot mixture to the pistachio mixture. Knead the two mixtures together until well combined. Flatten the mixture in the bowl. Using a sharp knife, cut the mixture into twelve wedges.
6. To shape the delights, dampen your hands with water, roll each wedge into a 2 x 1-inch log, and put them on a large plate. Roll each log in the reserved almond-coconut mixture until evenly coated on all sides. Store in an airtight container in the refrigerator or freezer.

Per serving: 265 calories, 7 g protein, 15 g fat (5 g sat), 32 g carbs, 46 mg sodium, 51 mg calcium, 5 g fiber

bliss balls

makes 12 balls, 4 servings

These little balls of confection are pure bliss. Made with dried fruit and nuts, they'll give you a shot of natural energy so you can maintain your endurance during work, play, or lovemaking.

3 tablespoons coconut water or water

1 teaspoon chia seeds

¾ cup walnuts

½ cup raisins

½ cup pitted soft dates

½ cup dried fruit (SUCH AS CHOPPED APRICOTS, CHERRIES, CRANBERRIES, CURRANTS, OR CHOPPED FIGS, OR A COMBINATION)

½ cup unsweetened shredded dried coconut, plus additional for coating

1½ tablespoons maca powder (OPTIONAL)

1 teaspoon vanilla extract

1 Put the coconut water and chia seeds in a small bowl and stir to combine. Let sit for 10 minutes to thicken into a gel.

2 Put the walnuts in a food processor and process until finely chopped. Transfer to a small plate.

3 Put the raisins, dates, and dried fruit in the food processor and process until finely chopped, 1 to 2 minutes. Add the chia seed mixture, reserved walnuts, coconut, optional maca powder, and vanilla extract and process until the mixture comes together to form a ball, 1 to 2 minutes.

4 Put some additional shredded coconut on a small plate. Dampen your hands with water, roll the fruit mixture into twelve one-inch balls, and then roll each ball in shredded coconut until evenly coated on all sides. Store in an airtight container in the refrigerator or freezer.

Per serving: 435 calories, 9 g protein, 32 g fat (17 g sat), 34 g carbs, 25 mg sodium, 47 mg calcium, 8 g fiber
Note: Analysis doesn't include additional coconut for coating.

cinnamon and vanilla almond kisses

makes 6 servings

Some people have a kitchen placard that states "Kiss the Cook!" You won't need to ask for kisses from your beloved when you offer these tantalizing almonds—you'll be showered with them!

1½ cups whole raw almonds
1 tablespoon vanilla extract
1½ teaspoons powdered sugar
1½ teaspoons ground cinnamon

1. Preheat the oven to 375 degrees F. Line a baking sheet with parchment paper or a silicone baking mat.
2. Arrange the almonds in a single layer on the lined baking sheet. Bake for 5 to 7 minutes, until the almonds are lightly toasted and fragrant.
3. Immediately transfer the almonds to a medium bowl. Add the vanilla extract (it will sizzle a bit) and stir to evenly coat the almonds.
4. Put the powdered sugar and cinnamon in a small bowl and stir to combine. Sprinkle over the almonds and gently toss until they're evenly coated. Store in an airtight container at room temperature.

turn-ons Replace the almonds with your favorite nuts, such as cashews, pecans, or walnuts.

CHAI ALMOND KISSES: Decrease the amount of cinnamon to ¾ teaspoon and add ½ teaspoon of ground cardamom and ¼ teaspoon of ground ginger to the powdered sugar.

Per serving: 148 calories, 5 g protein, 11 g fat (1 g sat), 6 g carbs, 1 mg sodium, 70 mg calcium, 3 g fiber

cocoa-coated cashews

makes 6 servings

These chocolate-dipped and cocoa-coated morsels can be enjoyed by the handful or used to top nondairy ice cream. Chocolate is inextricably intertwined with romance. It contains phenylethylamine, a compound known as the "love drug" because it creates a brain buzz that's similar to being in love.

1½ cups raw cashews
¾ cup vegan chocolate chips
1 tablespoon plain or vanilla nondairy milk
½ teaspoon vanilla extract
1½ tablespoons cacao powder or unsweetened cocoa powder

1. Preheat the oven to 375 degrees F. Line a baking sheet with parchment paper or a silicone baking mat.
2. Arrange the cashews in a single layer on the lined baking sheet. Bake for 5 to 7 minutes, until golden brown and fragrant. Let cool completely.
3. Put the chocolate chips, milk, and vanilla extract in a medium bowl and microwave for 1 to 2 minutes to melt the chips. Alternatively, put in a double boiler over medium-low heat until the chips are melted.
4. Add the cashews to the chocolate mixture and stir until evenly coated.
5. Using a slotted spoon or fork, remove the cashews one at a time from the chocolate and put them back on the lined baking sheet in a single layer, making sure they don't touch. Set aside the remaining melted chocolate. Refrigerate the coated cashews for 15 minutes. Repeat the chocolate coating and refrigerating procedure. (Double-dipping the cashews in the chocolate will create a thick layer.)
6. Put the cacao powder in a medium bowl. Add the chocolate-covered cashews and gently toss until evenly coated. Store in an airtight container in the refrigerator.

turn-ons Replace the cashews with your favorite nuts, such as almonds, hazelnuts, or pecans.

Per serving: 313 calories, 7 g protein, 22 g fat (8 g sat), 25 g carbs, 24 mg sodium, 62 mg calcium, 2 g fiber

santa fe trail mix

makes 8 servings

If you adore crunchy snacks and the smoky flavors of Southwestern cuisine, you'll find this colorful trail mix addictively good. Mix up a batch and your lover will literally be eating out of your hand.

- ½ teaspoon chili powder or chipotle chile powder
- ½ teaspoon garlic powder
- ½ teaspoon ground coriander
- ½ teaspoon ground cumin
- ½ teaspoon dried oregano
- ½ teaspoon smoked or sweet paprika
- 1 tablespoon lime juice
- 1½ teaspoons olive oil
- 1½ teaspoons reduced-sodium tamari or coconut aminos
- ½ cup mini pretzel nuggets, sticks, or twists
- ⅓ cup whole raw almonds
- ⅓ cup raw pecans
- ⅓ cup raw pumpkin seeds
- ¼ cup pine nuts
- ⅓ cup coarsely chopped dried mango
- ⅓ cup date pieces covered with oat flour
- ⅓ cup dried goji berries

1. Preheat the oven to 350 degrees F. Line a baking sheet with parchment paper or a silicone baking mat.
2. Put the chili powder, garlic powder, coriander, cumin, oregano, and paprika in a small bowl and stir to combine.
3. Put the lime juice, oil, and tamari in a medium bowl and stir to combine. Add the pretzels, almonds, pecans, pumpkin seeds, and pine nuts and stir to combine. Sprinkle the spice mixture over the top and stir until the pretzels and nuts are evenly coated.
4. Transfer to the lined baking sheet and spread into a single layer with a silicone spatula. Bake for 10 to 15 minutes, until the mixture is lightly toasted and fragrant. Let cool completely.
5. Transfer the cooled mixture to a medium bowl. Add the mango, dates, and goji berries and stir to combine. Store in an airtight container at room temperature.

Per serving: 214 calories, 6 g protein, 13 g fat (1 g sat), 23 g carbs, 251 mg sodium, 35 mg calcium, 3 g fiber

lemon-herb roasted chickpeas

makes 4 servings

Roasting chickpeas magically transforms them into crunchy munchables. They're perfect for popping into your (or your lover's) mouth, especially after a romantic interlude.

1 can (15 OUNCES) **chickpeas, drained and rinsed**

1 tablespoon lemon juice

2 teaspoons agave nectar or maple syrup

2 teaspoons olive oil (OPTIONAL)

1½ teaspoons nutritional yeast flakes

1½ teaspoons Italian seasoning, or ½ teaspoon each dried basil, oregano, and rosemary

1½ teaspoons garlic powder

½ teaspoon smoked or sweet paprika

1. Put the chickpeas on a clean kitchen towel or paper towels and let air-dry for 10 minutes.
2. Preheat the oven to 425 degrees F. Line a baking sheet with parchment paper or a silicone baking mat.
3. Put the lemon juice, agave nectar, optional oil, nutritional yeast, Italian seasoning, garlic powder, and paprika in a small bowl and stir to combine. Add the chickpeas and stir until evenly coated.
4. Transfer to the lined baking sheet and spread into a single layer with a silicone spatula. Bake for 25 to 30 minutes, shaking the pan every 10 minutes to ensure even baking, until the chickpeas are golden brown, dry, and slightly crunchy.

CHILE-LIME ROASTED CHICKPEAS: Replace the lemon juice with 1 tablespoon of lime juice. Replace the olive oil with 1 teaspoon of reduced-sodium tamari or coconut aminos and 1 teaspoon of toasted sesame oil. Replace the Italian seasoning with ½ teaspoon of chili powder, ½ teaspoon of ground cumin, and ¼ teaspoon of chipotle chile powder or cayenne.

Per serving: 147 calories, 9 g protein, 2 g fat (0.3 g sat), 25 g carbs, 9 mg sodium, 53 mg calcium, 7 g fiber

fruit-n-nut crackers

makes 48 crackers

Both almond flour and almond meal are combined with sunflower seeds and dried currants to create these sweet and nutty crackers. Serve them plain or topped with vegan cheese. They pair quite well with a glass of wine.

- 1 cup blanched almond flour
- 1 cup almond meal
- 1 tablespoon dried basil or dried thyme
- ¾ teaspoon sea salt
- ¼ cup water
- 1½ tablespoons sunflower oil or other oil
- ¼ cup coarsely chopped raw sunflower seeds
- 2 tablespoons dried currants

1. Preheat the oven to 300 degrees F. Line a baking sheet with parchment paper or a silicone baking mat.
2. Put the almond flour, almond meal, basil, and salt in a medium bowl and stir to combine.
3. Add the water and oil and stir to combine. Add the sunflower seeds and currants and stir until the mixture comes together to form a soft dough.
4. Transfer the dough to the lined baking sheet. Put another sheet of parchment paper or a silicone baking mat on top of the dough. Using a rolling pin, roll the dough into a 12 x 9-inch rectangle, about ⅛-inch thick.
5. Remove the top sheet of parchment paper. Using a sharp knife or pizza cutter, cut the dough into 1½-inch squares.
6. Bake for 18 to 22 minutes, until the crackers feel dry and are lightly browned around the edges. Watch closely during the last 2 minutes of baking to avoid burning. Let cool completely on the baking sheet. Store in an airtight container at room temperature or in the refrigerator.

turn-ons Replace the dried currants with 2 tablespoons of finely chopped dried cranberries, raisins, or soft dates.

SUPER SEED CRACKERS: Omit the dried basil and currants. Decrease the amount of chopped sunflower seeds to 2 tablespoons, and add 2 tablespoons each of hemp seeds, sesame seeds, and coarsely chopped raw pumpkin seeds.

Per 4 crackers: 49 calories, 1 g protein, 5 g fat (0.4 g sat), 1 g carbs, 118 mg sodium, 7 mg calcium, 1 g fiber

artichoke pâté

makes 4 servings

Artichokes are often coupled with lemons because their flavors complement each other and the lemon juice helps prevent the artichokes from turning brown. For this opulent pâté, artichokes carouse with almonds and pine nuts to create a spread you'll be proud to serve on the buffet table or in the boudoir.

½ cup whole raw almonds, soaked in water for at least 1 hour and drained
2 tablespoons pine nuts
¾ cup canned or thawed frozen artichoke hearts, quartered
2 tablespoons water
Zest and juice of ½ lemon (ABOUT 1½ TEASPOONS ZEST AND 2 TABLESPOONS JUICE)
1 tablespoon nutritional yeast flakes
1 tablespoon minced garlic
Sea salt

1 Squeeze each almond between your thumb and forefinger to remove the skin. Put the almonds and pine nuts in a food processor and process until finely ground. Scrape down the container with a silicone spatula.

2 Add the artichoke hearts, water, lemon zest and juice, nutritional yeast, and garlic and process until smooth. Season with salt to taste and process for 15 seconds longer. Store in an airtight container in the refrigerator.

Per serving: 136 calories, 5 g protein, 9 g fat (1 g sat), 10 g carbs, 295 mg sodium, 68 mg calcium, 5 g fiber
Note: Analysis doesn't include sea salt to taste.

kalamata olive hummus

makes 6 servings

Making hummus is a bit like making love—a little experimenting can have surprisingly delightful results. In this sophisticated version of traditional hummus, salty kalamata olives and sweet-and-tangy balsamic vinegar team up to create a spectacular contrast of flavors.

½ cup pitted kalamata olives
1 can (15 OUNCES) chickpeas, drained and rinsed
4 large cloves garlic
2 tablespoons balsamic vinegar
2 tablespoons lemon juice
2 tablespoons tahini
½ teaspoon ground cumin
Sea salt
Freshly ground black pepper
Sweet or smoked paprika (OPTIONAL)

1. Put the olives in a food processor and pulse until coarsely chopped. Put half the olives in a medium bowl and set aside.
2. Add the chickpeas and garlic to the food processor and process for 1 minute.
3. Add the vinegar, lemon juice, tahini, and cumin and process until smooth. Scrape down the container with a silicone spatula and process for 15 seconds longer.
4. Add the hummus to the reserved olives and stir until well combined. Season with salt and pepper to taste. Transfer to a storage container and sprinkle paprika over the top if desired. Store in an airtight container in the refrigerator.

Per serving: 124 calories, 5 g protein, 5 g fat (1 g sat), 15 g carbs, 108 mg sodium, 57 mg calcium, 5 g fiber
Note: Analysis doesn't include sea salt or freshly ground black pepper to taste.

smoked cheddar cheese ball

makes 4 servings

Break open the crackers or crostini and get this party started! A cheese ball always signals a good time. This sultry ball of cashew Cheddar is everything you want in a party animal—rich and smooth, with just a hint of smoke and spice.

1 cup raw cashews, soaked in water for at least 1 hour and drained
½ red bell pepper, diced
¼ cup nutritional yeast flakes
2 tablespoons lemon juice
1 teaspoon Dijon mustard
½ teaspoon garlic powder
½ teaspoon onion powder
½ teaspoon smoked or sweet paprika
½ teaspoon sea salt
⅛ teaspoon chipotle chile powder, cayenne, or hot sauce
⅓ cup pecans or walnuts, toasted and coarsely chopped

1. To make the cheese, put the cashews, bell pepper, nutritional yeast, lemon juice, mustard, garlic powder, onion powder, paprika, salt, and chile powder in a food processor and process until smooth. Scrape down the container with a silicone spatula and process for 15 seconds longer.

2. Have ready an eight-inch (or longer) sheet of plastic wrap. Put the cheese in the center of the plastic wrap, gently enclose the cheese with it, then use your hands to shape it into a ball. Refrigerate for at least 4 hours.

3. Remove the plastic wrap and put the cheese ball on a plate. Press the pecans into the ball until it's evenly coated on all sides. Cover the cheese ball with clean plastic wrap and refrigerate until ready to serve. Serve cold or room temperature.

turn-ons For a mild Cheddar taste, use sweet paprika and omit the chipotle chile powder.

Per serving: 307 calories, 11 g protein, 23 g fat (3 g sat), 19 g carbs, 86 mg sodium, 34 mg calcium, 5 g fiber

whoo-pea guacamole with baked tortilla chips

makes 4 servings

Excluding you, there's nothing more succulent than a perfectly ripe avocado. For this luxurious guacamole, green peas are added to reduce the fat content, so you can indulge to your heart's content. They not only add a touch of sweetness, but they also help retain the dip's vibrant green color.

4 (6-INCH) corn tortillas
1 avocado
1 cup frozen peas, thawed
1 jalapeño chile or serrano chile, seeded and finely diced
2 large cloves garlic, minced
Juice of ½ lime (ABOUT 1 TABLESPOON)
1½ teaspoons nutritional yeast flakes
½ teaspoon chili powder, or ¼ teaspoon hot sauce
¼ cup finely diced tomatoes
2 tablespoons finely diced red or yellow onion
2 tablespoons chopped fresh cilantro
Sea salt
Freshly ground black pepper

1. To make the tortilla chips, preheat the oven to 350 degrees F. Line a baking sheet with parchment paper or a silicone baking mat.
2. Stack the tortillas on top of each other, then cut into six wedges. Arrange the wedges in a single layer on the lined baking sheet.
3. Bake for 8 to 10 minutes, until the chips are crisp. Watch closely during the last 2 minutes of baking time to avoid burning.
4. To make the guacamole, put the avocado, peas, chile, garlic, lime juice, nutritional yeast, and chili powder in a food processor and process until smooth. Scrape down the container with a silicone spatula and process for 15 seconds longer.
5. Transfer to a small bowl. Add the tomatoes, onion, and cilantro and stir to combine. Season with salt and pepper to taste. Serve the guacamole with the warm or room temperature tortilla chips. Store leftover tortilla chips in an airtight container at room temperature. Store leftover guacamole in an airtight container in the refrigerator.

Per serving: 196 calories, 5 g protein, 10 g fat (2 g sat), 22 g carbs, 72 mg sodium, 26 mg calcium, 8 g fiber
Note: Analysis doesn't include sea salt or freshly ground black pepper to taste.

papaya-pineapple salsa

makes 6 servings

Juicy papaya and pineapple are the stars of this unique salsa. Scoop it up with Baked Tortilla Chips (page 151), your favorite store-bought tortilla chips, or just a spoon. It also makes a terrific topper for burritos, salads, and beans of any hue.

1 papaya, peeled, seeded, and diced
½ cup canned or thawed frozen pineapple tidbits
¾ cup diced red bell pepper
½ cup diced red onion
¼ cup chopped fresh cilantro, lightly packed
1 jalapeño chile, seeded and finely diced
Juice of 1 lime (ABOUT 2 TABLESPOONS)
1 tablespoon minced garlic
Sea salt
Freshly ground black pepper

1. Put the papaya, pineapple, bell pepper, onion, cilantro, chile, lime juice, and garlic in a medium bowl and stir to combine.
2. Season with salt and pepper to taste. Store leftover salsa in an airtight container in the refrigerator.

MANGO-PINEAPPLE SALSA: Replace the papaya with 2 mangoes, peeled, pitted, and diced.

Per serving: 40 calories, 1 g protein, 0 g fat (0 g sat), 10 g carbs, 6 mg sodium, 19 mg calcium, 2 g fiber
Note: Analysis doesn't include sea salt or freshly ground black pepper to taste.

hot artichoke and spinach dip

makes 6 servings

This ever-popular dip gets a vegan makeover that transforms it from good to phenomenal. It's moist, steamy, and bubbling—just like you and your main squeeze. Serve it hot, chaperoned by thinly sliced bread, crackers, or crudités to keep your urge to devour it all at once under control.

⅓ cup finely diced yellow onion
1 teaspoon olive oil
2 cups finely chopped baby spinach, lightly packed
1½ tablespoons minced garlic
1 can (14 OUNCES) artichoke hearts packed in water, drained and chopped
1⅓ cups plain unsweetened nondairy milk
Zest and juice of 1 lemon (ABOUT 1 TABLESPOON ZEST AND ¼ CUP JUICE)
3 tablespoons nutritional yeast flakes
2 tablespoons tapioca starch
1 teaspoon Dijon mustard
1 teaspoon dried basil
½ teaspoon sea salt
½ teaspoon crushed red pepper flakes
¼ teaspoon ground black pepper
⅔ cup shredded vegan mozzarella cheese
Smoked or sweet paprika

1. Preheat the oven to 400 degrees F. Lightly oil an 8-inch round or square baking pan or mist it with cooking spray.
2. Put the onion and oil in a large cast-iron or nonstick skillet and cook over medium-high heat, stirring occasionally, for 3 minutes.
3. Add the spinach and garlic and cook, stirring occasionally, until the spinach is tender, 2 to 3 minutes. Stir in the artichoke hearts. Transfer to the prepared baking pan.
4. Put the milk, lemon zest and juice, nutritional yeast, tapioca starch, mustard, basil, salt, red pepper flakes, and pepper in a blender and process until smooth. Scrape down the container with a silicone spatula and process for 15 seconds longer.
5. Add the milk mixture and cheese to the baking pan and stir to combine. Sprinkle a little paprika over the top.
6. Bake for 25 to 30 minutes, or until the dip is hot and bubbly around the edges.

Per serving: 112 calories, 6 g protein, 3 g fat (0.4 g sat), 19 g carbs, 306 mg sodium, 146 mg calcium, 6 g fiber
Note: Analysis doesn't include smoked paprika to garnish.

crispy buffalo cauliflower with ranch dressing

makes 4 servings

Cauliflower florets are dunked in a spicy batter, coated with a tongue-tingling breading, and then baked until golden brown and crispy. To offset the fiery edge of these scintillating morsels, plunge them into the cooling ranch dressing.

RANCH DRESSING

- ¾ cup plain unsweetened soy milk or other nondairy milk
- 2 tablespoons chopped fresh parsley
- 1 tablespoon cider vinegar
- 1 tablespoon nutritional yeast flakes
- 1½ teaspoons chia seeds
- ½ teaspoon dried dill weed
- ½ teaspoon dried thyme
- ½ teaspoon garlic powder
- ½ teaspoon onion powder

BATTER AND CAULIFLOWER

- ½ cup plain unsweetened soy milk or other nondairy milk
- ¼ cup blanched almond flour
- ¼ cup cornstarch
- 2 tablespoons hot sauce
- 1½ teaspoons cider vinegar
- 1½ teaspoons chili powder
- ½ teaspoon garlic powder
- ½ teaspoon sea salt
- ½ teaspoon ground black pepper
- 4 cups small cauliflower florets

BREADING

- ½ cup blanched almond flour
- ⅓ cup chickpea flour
- 2 tablespoons cornstarch
- 1 tablespoon nutritional yeast flakes
- 1½ teaspoons chili powder
- 1 teaspoon garlic powder
- 1 teaspoon onion powder
- 1 teaspoon chipotle chile powder or cayenne
- ½ teaspoon sea salt

1 To make the ranch dressing, put all the ingredients in a blender and process until smooth. Scrape down the container with a silicone spatula and let sit for 10 minutes. Process again for 15 seconds to break up any clumps of chia seeds. Transfer to an airtight container and refrigerate for 30 minutes to let the dressing thicken.

2 To make the batter, put the milk, almond flour, cornstarch, hot sauce, vinegar, chili powder, garlic powder, salt, and pepper in a large bowl and whisk to form a thick batter. Add the cauliflower and stir until evenly coated. Let marinate for 15 minutes, stirring every 5 minutes.

3 Preheat the oven to 450 degrees F. Line a baking sheet with parchment paper or a silicone baking mat.

4 To make the breading, put all the ingredients in a large ziplock bag or container with a tight-fitting lid and shake until well combined. Add the cauliflower to the bag and shake until evenly coated.

5 Arrange the cauliflower in a single layer on the lined baking sheet. Lightly drizzle a little olive oil over the cauliflower or mist it with cooking spray. Bake for 25 to 30 minutes, until the cauliflower is golden brown and crispy. Serve hot, with the ranch dressing on the side.

Per serving: 213 calories, 11 g protein, 6 g fat (1 g sat), 32 g carbs, 750 mg sodium, 72 mg calcium, 7 g fiber

cucumber canapés with red pepper spread

makes 4 servings

Finger foods are sexy without even trying. Among the most mouthwatering finger foods are canapés, which are small pieces of bread, pastry, or crackers covered with a savory topping. For this version, thick slices of cucumber are used instead of bread as the sturdy base for an impressive spread made with red peppers and cashews.

⅔ cup diced red bell pepper
2 large cloves garlic
1 tablespoon lemon juice
1 tablespoon water
½ cup raw cashews or pine nuts, soaked in water for at least 1 hour and drained
2 tablespoons nutritional yeast flakes
½ teaspoon smoked or sweet paprika
⅛ teaspoon cayenne or hot sauce
Sea salt
1 large cucumber, cut into 16 thick slices
Fresh parsley or dill sprigs

1 To make the spread, put the bell pepper, garlic, lemon juice, and water in a food processor and process until finely chopped, about 1 minute. Scrape down the container with a silicone spatula.

2 Add the cashews, nutritional yeast, paprika, and cayenne and process until smooth. Season with salt to taste and process for 15 seconds longer.

3 To assemble the canapés, arrange the cucumber in a single layer on a large plate or platter. Top each slice with 1 tablespoon of the spread. Garnish with parsley sprigs. Serve immediately.

CUCUMBER CANAPÉS WITH SUN-DRIED TOMATO SPREAD: Omit the red bell pepper. When soaking the cashews, add 3 whole sun-dried tomatoes (not packed in oil).

Per serving: 137 calories, 6 g protein, 8 g fat (2 g sat), 13 g carbs, 8 mg sodium, 29 mg calcium, 3 g fiber
Note: Analysis doesn't include sea salt to taste or parsley to garnish.

a little something on the side

When it comes to work or play, a little something on the side can fill a void or round things out. When it comes to meals, a little something on the side can fill an empty spot on your plate. Little somethings are more than passing flings—they're often the best part of the day or meal or whatnot. In fact, several of them served together can become the main attraction.

citrus-scented asparagus

makes 2 servings

Eating with your fingers is incredibly sensual, especially when you're feeding the object of your affections. If that's your penchant, cook these lemony asparagus only until they're crisp-tender, because a limp spear simply won't cut it.

1 pound asparagus, trimmed
1½ teaspoons olive oil
Zest and juice of 1 lemon (ABOUT 1 TABLESPOON ZEST AND ¼ CUP JUICE)
2 tablespoons chopped fresh parsley
1 tablespoon minced garlic
Sea salt
Freshly ground black pepper

1. Put the asparagus and oil in a large cast-iron or nonstick skillet and cook over medium heat, stirring occasionally, for 3 minutes.
2. Add the lemon zest and juice, parsley, and garlic and cook, stirring occasionally, until as tender as you like, 2 to 3 minutes. Season with salt and pepper to taste. Serve hot.

turn-ons For an oil-free version, replace the olive oil with 1 to 2 tablespoons of water or vegetable broth. For a spicy version, sprinkle crushed red pepper flakes over the finished dish.

Per serving: 84 calories, 5 g protein, 4 g fat (1 g sat), 10 g carbs, 13 mg sodium, 62 mg calcium, 5 g fiber
Note: Analysis doesn't include sea salt or freshly ground black pepper to taste.

steamed artichokes with saffron-almond dipping sauce

makes 4 servings

Eating an artichoke is a carnal event. If you've never indulged, here's how to do it. Peel off the outer petals one at a time, starting at the base. Dip the pulpy portion into the dipping sauce and pull the petal through your teeth to remove the soft, succulent flesh. Discard the remaining petal. Continue until all the petals have been removed. Spoon out the fuzzy center (called the choke) at the base and discard it. The bottom, or heart, of the artichoke is entirely edible. Cut it into small pieces and dip them into the sauce. Pure heaven!

ARTICHOKES

4 large globe artichokes

1 lemon, cut in half

SAFFRON-ALMOND DIPPING SAUCE

Pinch saffron threads

3 tablespoons hot water

1 medium shallot, finely diced, or ½ cup finely diced yellow onion

¼ cup sliced raw almonds

2 large cloves garlic

1½ tablespoons lemon juice

1 cup plain unsweetened nondairy yogurt

Sea salt

Freshly ground black pepper

1. To prep each artichoke for steaming, snap off a few of the tough lower leaves (pull them downward toward the stem) and discard. Using a serrated knife, cut off the stem, then trim about one inch off the top of the artichoke and discard. Using kitchen scissors, snip off the sharp thorny tips of the petals and discard. Rub the cut surfaces of the artichoke with the lemon to prevent discoloration.

2. Put a collapsible steamer basket or steamer rack into a large saucepan. Add enough water to just touch the bottom of the collapsible steamer, or make the water two inches deep if using a rack. Cover the saucepan and bring to a boil over medium heat.

3. Put the artichokes in the steamer and steam until the hearts can be easily pierced with the tip of a knife and the inner leaves pull out easily, 25 to 35 minutes. Transfer to a large plate or platter.

4. While the artichokes are steaming, prepare the dipping sauce. Put the saffron in a small bowl and add 1 tablespoon of the hot water. Let sit for 10 minutes to soften the saffron.

5. Put the remaining 2 tablespoons of hot water in a small saucepan. Add the shallot, almonds, and garlic and cook over medium heat, stirring occasionally, until the shallot is tender and all the water has evaporated, 3 to 5 minutes.

6. Transfer to a food processor. Add the saffron mixture and lemon juice and process until smooth. Scrape down the container with a silicone spatula. Add the yogurt and process for 30 seconds. Season with salt and pepper to taste and process for 15 seconds longer.

7. Serve the artichokes hot or room temperature, with the dipping sauce on the side.

turn-ons If you don't have access to saffron, omit it. Instead, add a pinch of ground turmeric directly to the blender with the shallot. If you prefer, you can skip the sauce altogether and simply serve the artichokes with a side of melted vegan butter for dipping.

Per serving: 208 calories, 7 g protein, 5 g fat (1 g sat), 38 g carbs, 14 mg sodium, 160 mg calcium, 5 g fiber
Note: Analysis doesn't include sea salt or freshly ground black pepper to taste.

steamed vegetables infused with lemon and ginger

makes 4 servings

One of the healthiest ways to cook vegetables is by steaming them until they're crisp-tender. Adding lemon and ginger to the cooking water will subtly infuse their flavors into the vegetables. Serve them up in the nude (the veggies, not you, you naughty tempter!) or take them skinny dipping with your favorite sauce.

1 lemon, cut in half

1 (1-INCH) **piece fresh ginger, thinly sliced**

1½ cups small broccoli florets

1½ cups small cauliflower florets

1 cup halved baby carrots, or 1 cup diagonally sliced carrots

1 cup asparagus, trimmed and cut in half diagonally

1 cup snap peas or pea pods

Sea salt

Freshly ground black pepper or lemon pepper

1. Leave one lemon half intact. Cut the other half into 4 wedges and set aside.
2. Put a collapsible steamer basket or steamer rack into a large saucepan. Add enough water to just touch the bottom of the collapsible steamer, or make the water two inches deep if using a rack. Put the intact lemon half and ginger into the water. Cover the saucepan and bring to a boil over medium heat.
3. Steam the vegetables in batches until crisp-tender. The broccoli and cauliflower will take 5 to 7 minutes, the carrots 3 to 5 minutes, and the asparagus and snap peas 2 to 3 minutes.
4. Transfer the steamed vegetables to a large bowl and stir to combine. Alternatively, arrange the vegetables in rows or in a circle on a large plate or platter. Season with salt and pepper to taste.
5. Squeeze a lemon wedge over each serving. Serve hot or room temperature.

turn-ons To take your veggies skinny dipping, try Cheesy Sauce (page 184), Creamy Hemp Seed Dressing (page 125), or Creamy Saffron-Almond Dipping Sauce (page 158).

Per serving: 55 calories, 4 g protein, 0 g fat (0 g sat), 11 g carbs, 62 mg sodium, 36 mg calcium, 4 g fiber
Note: Analysis doesn't include sea salt or freshly ground black pepper to taste.

roman artichoke-and-asparagus bake

makes 4 servings

Rome is one of the most romantic cities in the world, and it provided the inspiration for this enticing side dish. Artichokes, asparagus, basil, garlic, olives, and tomatoes are common ingredients in Italian cuisine, and their colors and flavors complement each other like the perfect hookup on a dating site. This one's a keeper.

1 pound asparagus, trimmed and cut diagonally into 2-inch pieces

1 can (14 OUNCES) **artichoke hearts packed in water, drained and quartered**

1½ cups diced tomatoes

¾ cup pitted kalamata or black olives, quartered lengthwise

½ cup chopped fresh basil, lightly packed

1½ tablespoons minced garlic

1 tablespoon nutritional yeast flakes

½ teaspoon crushed red pepper flakes

½ teaspoon sea salt

¼ teaspoon ground black pepper

1. Preheat the oven to 425 degrees F. Lightly oil a 9-inch square baking pan or mist it with cooking spray.
2. Put all the ingredients in a large bowl and stir to combine. Transfer to the prepared baking pan.
3. Bake for 7 minutes. Remove from the oven and stir. Bake for 5 to 10 minutes longer, until all the vegetables are tender. Serve hot.

Per serving: 135 calories, 10 g protein, 4 g fat (1 g sat), 22 g carbs, 555 mg sodium, 106 mg calcium, 11 g fiber

baked potatoes topped with broccoli and cheese

makes 4 servings

Transform plain baked potatoes from ho-hum to yum by topping them with a cheesy sauce and tender broccoli florets. To save time, make the sauce while the potatoes are baking. Serve these sexy spuds as a side dish, or partner them with a salad for a filling lunch or dinner.

4 large russet potatoes
Sea salt
Freshly ground black pepper
2 cups bite-sized broccoli florets, cooked until tender
1 recipe Cheesy Sauce (PAGE 184)**, hot**

1. To cook the potatoes in the oven, preheat the oven to 400 degrees F. Line a baking sheet with parchment paper or a silicone baking mat. Using a fork, pierce each potato in several places on all sides and put them on the lined baking sheet. Bake for 40 to 45 minutes (turning them over after 25 minutes), until the potatoes are soft and can be easily squeezed. Alternatively, to cook the pierced potatoes in the microwave, put them in a pie pan or baking dish and microwave for 15 to 20 minutes, until the potatoes are soft.
2. Using a sharp knife, cut a slit down the length of each potato. Gently squeeze the sides toward the middle to open the potatoes, then put them on a large platter or on individual plates. Alternatively, cut each potato in half lengthwise and put them cut-side up on a platter or plate. Season each potato with salt and pepper to taste.
3. Top each potato with ⅓ to ½ cup of the sauce and ½ cup of the broccoli. Serve hot.

turn-ons Top each potato with 1 slice of Tempeh Bacon (page 116), coarsely chopped, or 1 tablespoon of Coconut Bacon (page 102).

Per serving: 473 calories, 16 g protein, 6 g fat (1 g sat), 82 g carbs, 410 mg sodium, 110 mg calcium, 13 g fiber
Note: Analysis doesn't include sea salt or freshly ground black pepper to taste.

ginger-braised carrots

makes 4 servings

Braising involves slowly cooking food in a tightly covered saucepan with a small amount of liquid. For this dish, carrots are braised in coconut water with fresh ginger and then finished with parsley and coconut oil. This recipe proves that sumptuous doesn't always mean complicated!

- **1 pound carrots, halved lengthwise and cut into 2-inch pieces, or 1 pound whole baby carrots**
- **⅔ cup coconut water**
- **1½ tablespoons peeled and grated fresh ginger**
- **⅓ cup chopped fresh parsley, lightly packed**
- **1½ teaspoons coconut oil or vegan butter** (OPTIONAL)
- **Sea salt**

1. Put the carrots, coconut water, and ginger in a large saucepan. Cover and cook over medium heat until the carrots are tender, 10 to 12 minutes.

2. Add the parsley and optional coconut oil and stir to combine. Season with salt to taste. Serve hot.

turn-ons For a richer-tasting dish, replace the coconut water with ⅔ cup of plain unsweetened coconut milk beverage or canned coconut milk.

GINGER-AND-MAPLE CANDIED CARROTS: After the carrots are tender, add 2 tablespoons of maple syrup to the saucepan and cook uncovered, stirring occasionally, until the liquid thickens into a glaze, 2 to 3 minutes.

Per serving: 57 calories, 1 g protein, 0 g fat (0 g sat), 14 g carbs, 93 mg sodium, 47 mg calcium, 3 g fiber
Note: Analysis doesn't include sea salt to taste.

bayou beans

makes 4 servings

The "holy trinity" of Cajun and Creole cooking is onion, celery, and bell pepper. It forms the foundation for almost every savory dish, including this one, which is a vegan spin on a classic New Orleans recipe. For an extra-hearty meal, especially after a little hanky-panky, serve the beans over warm cornbread or hot rice.

1 cup dried red beans or kidney beans, sorted and rinsed
⅔ cup diced yellow onion
⅔ cup diced celery
⅔ cup diced red or green bell pepper
1 tablespoon olive oil, or ¼ cup low-sodium vegetable broth or water
1 jalapeño chile, seeded and finely diced
1½ tablespoons minced garlic
1½ teaspoons chili powder
1 teaspoon dried oregano
1 teaspoon dried thyme
¼ teaspoon cayenne or chipotle chile powder
3½ cups water
1 bay leaf
3 Seitan Sausages (PAGE 114)**, coarsely chopped**
⅓ cup thinly sliced green onions
Sea salt
Freshly ground black pepper

1 Put the beans in a large saucepan or soup pot and cover with warm water. Let soak for 8 to 12 hours. Drain in a colander and set aside. Rinse the saucepan and reuse.

2 Put the onion, celery, bell pepper, and oil in the saucepan and cook over medium heat, stirring occasionally, for 5 minutes.

3 Add the chile, garlic, chili powder, oregano, thyme, and cayenne and cook, stirring occasionally, for 2 minutes.

4 Add the beans, water, and bay leaf and stir to combine. Bring to a boil over high heat. Cover, decrease the heat to low, and simmer until the beans are soft, about 1 hour.

5 Remove and discard the bay leaf. Add the sausages and green onions and cook, stirring occasionally, for 5 minutes. Season with salt and pepper to taste. Serve hot.

Per serving: 279 calories, 16 g protein, 7 g fat (2 g sat), 40 g carbs, 126 mg sodium, 107 mg calcium, 10 g fiber
Note: Analysis doesn't include sea salt or freshly ground black pepper to taste.

okra soycutash

makes 4 servings

In this revamped version of succotash, plump edamame stand in for the customary lima beans, and jalapeño chile and okra are added to the traditional mix of corn, bell pepper, and tomato. It's a Deep South favorite, and once you go deep, you'll never go back.

1 package (10 OUNCES) **frozen corn kernels**
1 package (10 OUNCES) **frozen sliced okra**
1 cup diced red bell pepper
⅔ cup diced tomatoes
⅔ cup frozen shelled edamame
½ cup low-sodium vegetable broth
1 jalapeño chile, cut in half lengthwise and thinly sliced
⅓ cup thinly sliced green onions
¼ cup chopped fresh parsley, lightly packed
1 tablespoon nutritional yeast flakes
1 teaspoon chili powder
1 teaspoon dried oregano
1 teaspoon dried thyme
¼ teaspoon cayenne or chipotle chile powder
Sea salt
Freshly ground black pepper

1 Put the corn, okra, bell pepper, tomatoes, edamame, broth, and chile in a large saucepan or nonstick skillet and stir to combine. Cover and cook over medium-high heat, stirring occasionally, until the vegetables are tender, 8 to 10 minutes.

2 Add the green onions, parsley, nutritional yeast, chili powder, oregano, thyme, and cayenne and cook, stirring occasionally, until the broth has evaporated, 1 to 2 minutes. Season with salt and pepper to taste. Serve hot.

Per serving: 289 calories, 19 g protein, 4 g fat (1 g sat), 58 g carbs, 44 mg sodium, 662 mg calcium, 22 g fiber
Note: Analysis doesn't include sea salt or freshly ground black pepper to taste.

roasted roots

makes 4 servings

It's not surprising that root vegetables, which grow deep in the ground, have an earthy flavor, but they have a hint of sweetness too. They release their natural sugars when they're oven-roasted, which makes them sweeter and even more captivating. A drizzle of balsamic vinegar further heightens their allure.

- 1 pound beets
- 1 pound root vegetables (SUCH AS PARSNIPS, RUTABAGAS, OR TURNIPS, OR A COMBINATION)
- ¼ cup low-sodium vegetable broth
- 1½ tablespoons olive oil
- 1 tablespoon nutritional yeast flakes
- 4 large cloves garlic, thinly sliced
- 2 teaspoons Italian seasoning, or ½ teaspoon each dried basil, oregano, and rosemary
- Sea salt
- Freshly ground black pepper
- 2 tablespoons balsamic vinegar

1. Preheat the oven to 400 degrees F. Line a baking sheet with parchment paper or a silicone baking mat.
2. Peel the beets and root vegetables if desired, then cut them into 1½-inch cubes or small wedges.
3. Put the broth, oil, nutritional yeast, garlic, and Italian seasoning in a large bowl and whisk to combine. Add the beets and root vegetables and stir until evenly coated. Transfer to the lined baking sheet and spread into a single layer.
4. Bake for 20 minutes. Remove from the oven, stir, and spread into a single layer again. Bake for 15 to 20 minutes longer, until the vegetables are tender and lightly browned around the edges.
5. Season with salt and pepper to taste. Drizzle the vinegar over the top and stir to combine. Serve hot.

Per serving: 197 calories, 5 g protein, 6 g fat (1 g sat), 34 g carbs, 105 mg sodium, 73 mg calcium, 9 g fiber
Note: Analysis doesn't include sea salt or freshly ground black pepper to taste.

tomatoes rockefeller

makes 4 servings

Oysters Rockefeller, a glitzy dish created in New Orleans in 1899, was named for millionaire John D. Rockefeller because the unfortunate oysters were topped with a money-colored green herb sauce. For this veganized version, large tomato halves hold a vibrant spinach-based filling topped with bread crumbs. Dig into these voluptuous beauties and feel like a millionaire!

- 2 large tomatoes
- ½ cup finely diced yellow onion, or 1 medium shallot, finely diced
- 1 tablespoon olive oil, or 2 to 3 tablespoons low-sodium vegetable broth or water
- 4 cups coarsely chopped baby spinach, lightly packed
- 1½ tablespoons minced garlic
- ¼ cup chopped fresh basil, lightly packed
- 2 tablespoons chopped fresh parsley
- 1 tablespoon nutritional yeast flakes
- ¼ teaspoon smoked or sweet paprika
- ¼ teaspoon sea salt
- ⅛ teaspoon ground black pepper
- ⅛ teaspoon ground nutmeg
- 2 tablespoons dry or fresh bread crumbs

1. Preheat the oven to 375 degrees F.
2. To prep the tomatoes, cut each tomato in half crosswise. Using your fingers, gently remove the seeds while keeping the tomato halves intact. Put the tomatoes in an 8-inch square baking dish cut-side up.
3. Put the onion and oil in a large cast-iron or nonstick skillet and cook over medium heat, stirring occasionally, for 3 minutes.
4. Add the spinach and garlic and cook, stirring occasionally, until the spinach is wilted, 2 to 3 minutes. Add the basil, parsley, nutritional yeast, paprika, salt, pepper, and nutmeg and stir to combine. Remove from the heat.
5. Evenly spoon the spinach mixture on top of each tomato half and sprinkle with the bread crumbs.
6. Bake for 15 to 20 minutes, until the tomatoes are slightly soft and the bread crumbs are lightly browned. Serve hot.

Per serving: 88 calories, 4 g protein, 4 g fat (1 g sat), 11 g carbs, 174 mg sodium, 62 mg calcium, 3 g fiber

quinoa with grapes and pistachios

makes 4 servings

Side dishes are capricious—they can be savory or sweet and served hot, room temperature, or even chilled. This one embodies that fanciful nature. Cooked quinoa is seasoned with a tantalizing dressing, then it's tossed with juicy grapes, cucumber, and pistachios.

1 cup white, red, or tricolor quinoa, rinsed
¾ cup apple juice
⅔ cup water
1 tablespoon peeled and grated fresh ginger
2 tablespoons red wine vinegar or cider vinegar
1 tablespoon toasted sesame oil
1 teaspoon agave nectar or maple syrup
½ teaspoon sea salt
¼ teaspoon ground black pepper
¼ teaspoon ground cinnamon
½ cup diced cucumber
½ cup halved red seedless grapes
½ cup halved white seedless grapes
½ cup raw or roasted pistachios
¼ cup thinly sliced green onions
¼ cup chopped fresh parsley, lightly packed

1. Put the quinoa, apple juice, water, and ginger in medium saucepan and stir to combine. Bring to a boil over high heat. Cover, decrease the heat to low, and cook until the quinoa is tender and all the liquid is absorbed, 15 to 18 minutes.
2. Fluff with a fork to loosen the grains. Let cool for 10 minutes, then fluff again. Transfer to a large bowl.
3. To make the dressing, put the vinegar, oil, agave nectar, salt, pepper, and cinnamon in a small bowl and whisk to combine. Pour over the quinoa and gently stir until evenly coated.
4. Add the cucumber, red grapes, white grapes, pistachios, green onions, and parsley and gently stir to combine. Serve warm, room temperature, or cold.

turn-ons To serve as a salad, double the dressing, add 2 cups of baby mixed greens or coarsely chopped leafy greens, and toss gently to combine.

Per serving: 272 calories, 8 g protein, 10 g fat (1 g sat), 40 g carbs, 339 mg sodium, 51 mg calcium, 5 g fiber

orange-scented couscous with apricots, cherries, and pine nuts

makes 4 servings

Couscous is lightly perfumed with a hint of orange, then combined with pink pickled onions, toasted pine nuts, and chewy dried fruit to add a pop of color and textural contrast to this winsome side dish.

1 cup water
Zest and juice of 1 orange (ABOUT 3 TABLESPOONS ZEST AND ½ CUP JUICE)
1 tablespoon peeled and grated fresh ginger
1 cup white or whole wheat couscous
1½ tablespoons white or red wine vinegar
1 tablespoon olive oil
½ cup diced red onion
⅓ cup pine nuts, toasted
⅓ cup coarsely chopped dried apricots
⅓ cup dried cherries or cranberries
⅓ cup chopped fresh parsley, lightly packed
Sea salt
Freshly ground black pepper

1. Put the water, orange zest and juice, and ginger in a medium saucepan. Bring to a boil over high heat. Add the couscous, cover, and remove from the heat. Let sit for 5 minutes to allow the couscous to absorb the liquid.
2. Fluff with a fork to loosen the grains. Add 1 tablespoon of the vinegar and the oil and gently stir to evenly coat the couscous. Transfer the couscous to a large bowl.
3. Rinse the saucepan and reuse. Fill the saucepan with one inch of water and bring to a boil over high heat. Add the onion and boil for 30 seconds. Drain in a colander and return the onion to the saucepan. Add the remaining ½ tablespoon of vinegar and stir to combine (this will turn the onion a vibrant pink).
4. Add the onion, pine nuts, apricots, cherries, and parsley to the couscous and gently stir to combine. Season with salt and pepper to taste. Serve warm, room temperature, or cold.

Per serving: 295 calories, 8 g protein, 12 g fat (1 g sat), 41 g carbs, 9 mg sodium, 26 mg calcium, 4 g fiber
Note: Analysis doesn't include sea salt or freshly ground black pepper to taste.

down-n-dirty rice

makes 4 servings

Dirty rice is a traditional Cajun dish that typically contains minced or ground meat along with spices and aromatic vegetables. This cheeky meatless version contains many of the customary components but uses mushrooms, nuts, and sunflower seeds to achieve that rich, time-honored flavor and color. Ready to get down and dirty?

- **2 cups water**
- **1 cup mixed rice and wild rice blend or long-grain brown rice, rinsed**
- **½ cup raw nuts** (SUCH AS ALMONDS, PECANS, OR WALNUTS, OR A COMBINATION)**, chopped**
- **2 tablespoons raw sunflower seeds, coarsely chopped**
- **1 cup finely diced button or cremini mushrooms**
- **½ cup finely diced yellow onion**
- **½ cup finely diced celery**
- **2 teaspoons olive oil, or ¼ cup low-sodium vegetable broth**
- **¼ cup thinly sliced green onions**
- **2 tablespoons minced garlic**
- **1½ teaspoons chili powder**
- **1½ teaspoons dried oregano**
- **1½ teaspoons dried thyme**
- **¼ teaspoon ground black pepper**
- **¼ teaspoon cayenne or hot sauce**
- **⅓ cup chopped fresh parsley, lightly packed**
- **1½ tablespoons reduced-sodium tamari or coconut aminos**

1. Put the water and rice in a medium saucepan and bring to a boil over high heat. Cover, decrease the heat to low, and cook until the rice is tender and the water is absorbed, 35 to 40 minutes. Remove from the heat.
2. While the rice is cooking, put the nuts and sunflower seeds in a large cast-iron or nonstick skillet and cook over medium heat, stirring occasionally, until lightly toasted and fragrant, 3 to 5 minutes. Transfer to a small plate and set aside.
3. Rinse the skillet and reuse. Put the mushrooms, onion, celery, and oil in the skillet and cook over medium-high heat, stirring occasionally, for 5 minutes. Add the green onions, garlic, chili powder, oregano, thyme, pepper, and cayenne and cook, stirring occasionally, until the vegetables are tender, 2 to 3 minutes. Remove from the heat.
4. Fluff the rice with a fork to loosen the grains and add it to the vegetables. Add the reserved nut mixture, parsley, and tamari and stir to combine. Serve hot.

DOWN-N-DIRTY CAULIFLOWER RICE: Replace the cooked rice with 3 cups packaged cauliflower rice. Alternatively, transform 1 medium head of cauliflower into rice-sized pieces by chopping it in a food processor or grating it by hand with a box grater.

Per serving: 293 calories, 8 g protein, 9 g fat (1 g sat), 46 g carbs, 292 mg sodium, 104 mg calcium, 4 g fiber

spiced and smashed sweet potatoes

makes 4 servings

Sweet potatoes are mashed with maple syrup, coconut oil, cinnamon, nutmeg, and vanilla, plus a shot of bourbon, to create this swoon-worthy side dish. Serve these sweeties in the buff or dress them in formal attire with the optional toppings. You'll be tipsy in love.

SPICED SWEET POTATOES

1½ pounds (4 TO 5 MEDIUM) sweet potatoes, peeled and cut into 2-inch cubes
2 tablespoons maple syrup
2 tablespoons bourbon
2 teaspoons coconut oil or vegan butter (OPTIONAL)
1½ teaspoons ground cinnamon
1 teaspoon vanilla extract
¼ teaspoon ground nutmeg

OPTIONAL TOPPINGS

⅓ cup pecans or pumpkin seeds, toasted and coarsely chopped
¼ cup unsweetened shredded dried coconut, toasted

1. Put the sweet potatoes in a large saucepan or soup pot and cover with water. Cook over medium-high heat until tender, 20 to 25 minutes. Reserve ⅓ cup of the cooking water. Drain the sweet potatoes in a colander.

2. Pour the reserved cooking water into the saucepan. Add the maple syrup, bourbon, optional coconut oil, cinnamon, vanilla extract, and nutmeg and stir to combine. Bring to a boil over medium heat. Remove from the heat.

3. Add the sweet potatoes to the saucepan. Using a potato masher, mash the sweet potatoes until smooth and creamy. Serve hot, garnished with one or both of the optional toppings.

Per serving: 249 calories, 3 g protein, 1 g fat (0.1 g sat), 55 g carbs, 16 mg sodium, 45 mg calcium, 8 g fiber
Note: Analysis doesn't include optional toppings.

farro with kale and pomegranate seeds

makes 4 servings

Farro is known as the mother of all grains because it's believed to be the original grain from which all others (barley, rice, rye, and wheat) were derived. It dates back over six thousand years to the Egyptians. If you like experimenting with unconventional grains (or anything else unconventional!), this dish will be right up your alley.

- 3 cups water
- 1 cup farro, rinsed
- 10 leaves lacinato kale, stemmed and cut into thin ribbons
- ½ cup diced red onion
- 1 tablespoon olive oil, or 2 to 3 tablespoons water
- 1 tablespoon minced garlic
- ½ cup chopped fresh parsley, lightly packed
- ⅓ cup golden raisins
- Juice of ½ lemon (ABOUT 2 TABLESPOONS)
- Sea salt
- Freshly ground black pepper
- ⅓ cup pomegranate seeds
- ⅓ cup sliced almonds, toasted

1. Put the water and farro in a medium saucepan and bring to a boil over high heat. Cover, decrease the heat to low, and cook until the farro is tender and all the water is absorbed, 30 to 40 minutes. Remove from the heat.
2. While the farro is cooking, put the kale, onion, and oil in a large cast-iron or nonstick skillet and cook over medium-high heat, stirring occasionally, for 5 minutes. Add the garlic and cook, stirring occasionally, until the kale is tender, 2 to 3 minutes. Remove from the heat.
3. Add the farro, parsley, raisins, and lemon juice and stir to combine. Season with salt and pepper to taste. Add the pomegranate seeds and almonds and stir to combine. Serve hot or room temperature.

turn-ons Replace the farro with 1 cup of wheat berries or spelt berries and increase the cooking time to 1 hour.

Per serving: 358 calories, 11 g protein, 9 g fat (1 g sat), 58 g carbs, 30 mg sodium, 133 mg calcium, 10 g fiber
Note: Analysis doesn't include sea salt or freshly ground black pepper to taste.

confetti coconut rice

makes 4 servings

This creamy rice dish is loaded with tropical flavor. It's bejeweled with black beans, bell peppers, green onions, and cilantro and crowned with a coconut garnish. Although it's a looker, it's got substance as well as beauty.

- 2 cups water
- 1 cup white or brown basmati rice, rinsed
- ¼ cup plain unsweetened coconut milk beverage or canned coconut milk
- Juice of ½ orange (ABOUT ¼ CUP)
- Juice of 1 lime (ABOUT 2 TABLESPOONS)
- 1 tablespoon minced garlic
- 1 tablespoon peeled and grated fresh ginger
- 1½ teaspoons toasted sesame oil or coconut oil, melted
- ¼ teaspoon crushed red pepper flakes
- 1 can (15 OUNCES) black beans, drained and rinsed
- ½ cup diced orange or yellow bell pepper
- ½ cup diced red bell pepper
- ¼ cup thinly sliced green onions
- ¼ cup chopped fresh cilantro or parsley, lightly packed
- Sea salt
- Freshly ground black pepper
- ¼ cup unsweetened coconut chips, toasted, or 2 tablespoons unsweetened shredded dried coconut, toasted

1. Put the water and rice in a medium saucepan and bring to a boil over high heat. Cover, decrease the heat to low, and cook until the rice is tender and all the water is absorbed, about 20 minutes for white basmati rice or 30 minutes for brown basmati rice. Remove from the heat.

2. Fluff with a fork to loosen the grains. Add the milk, orange juice, lime juice, garlic, ginger, oil, and red pepper flakes and gently stir to combine.

3. Add the beans, orange bell pepper, red bell pepper, green onions, and cilantro and gently stir to combine. Season with salt and pepper to taste. Scatter the coconut over the top. Serve hot, warm, or room temperature.

Per serving: 482 calories, 12 g protein, 19 g fat (15 g sat), 66 g carbs, 14 mg sodium, 48 mg calcium, 8 g fiber
Note: Analysis doesn't include sea salt or freshly ground black pepper to taste.

main event

Sure, heavy petting with drinks and appetizers is pleasurable when schedules are light. But when hunger hits like a lightning bolt, there's little interest in fooling around. It's impossible to resist the urge to dive right into the heart of the action. The recipes in this section will get the sparks flying in no time flat. They're varied (because no one wants to get into a rut) and appeal to a range of tastes and appetites. As a bonus, they all make four servings, which means there will be plenty of leftovers to enjoy when canoodling takes priority over cooking.

pita pizza party

makes 4 servings

Forget takeout when it's so easy to make pizza at home using ready-made pita bread. These sublime pies make a welcome post-amoré snack. You'll be licking your fingers . . . and your companion's too.

- 4 (6-INCH) pita breads
- 12 tablespoons jarred marinara sauce
- 1 cup coarsely chopped baby spinach, lightly packed
- 6 tablespoons sliced or diced red or yellow onion
- 6 tablespoons sliced or diced red or orange bell pepper
- 8 artichoke hearts, quartered, or 4 button or cremini mushrooms, thinly sliced
- 1 cup shredded vegan mozzarella cheese, or ¾ cup Cheesy Sauce (PAGE 184)
- 4 teaspoons nutritional yeast flakes
- Freshly ground black pepper
- Crushed red pepper flakes (OPTIONAL)

1. Preheat the oven to 425 degrees F. Line a baking sheet with parchment paper or a silicone baking mat.
2. Put the pita breads on the baking sheet and spread the sauce evenly over them. Scatter the spinach, onion, bell pepper, and artichoke hearts over the sauce. Sprinkle with the cheese and nutritional yeast. Season with pepper and optional red pepper flakes to taste.
3. Bake for 8 to 10 minutes, until the pita breads are lightly browned around the edges and the cheese is melted. Cut each pizza into four wedges. Serve hot.

Per serving: 425 calories, 20 g protein, 5 g fat (1 g sat), 85 g carbs, 901 mg sodium, 260 mg calcium, 24 g fiber
Note: Analysis doesn't include freshly ground black pepper to taste.

veggie paella

makes 4 servings

Spain is famous for its paella, which is a saffron-infused rice dish made with an assortment of seafood and vegetables. In this recipe, the seafood is left in the sea and a colorful blend of mushrooms, artichoke hearts, bell pepper, peas, tomatoes, and olives is used instead.

2 cups low-sodium vegetable broth
½ teaspoon sea salt
¼ teaspoon ground black pepper
¼ teaspoon saffron threads or ground turmeric
⅔ cup halved and thinly sliced button or cremini mushrooms
½ cup diced yellow onion
½ cup diced red bell pepper
1½ tablespoons olive oil
1 cup long-grain white rice, rinsed
½ cup diced tomatoes
1 tablespoon minced garlic
½ cup artichoke hearts, quartered
½ cup frozen peas, thawed, or ½ cup pea pods, cut in half diagonally
⅓ cup pitted kalamata or black olives, sliced
¼ cup chopped fresh parsley, lightly packed
1 tablespoon lemon juice

1. Put the broth, salt, pepper, and saffron in a small saucepan and bring to a simmer over low heat.
2. Put the mushrooms, onion, bell pepper, and oil in a large cast-iron or nonstick skillet and cook over medium heat, stirring occasionally, for 5 minutes. Add the rice and stir until evenly coated. Add the tomatoes and garlic and cook, stirring constantly, for 2 minutes.
3. Add the simmering broth to the rice mixture and stir to combine. Bring to a boil over high heat. Cover, decrease the heat to low, and cook until the rice is tender and all the water is absorbed, 15 to 20 minutes. Remove from the heat.
4. Fluff with a fork to loosen the grains. Add the artichokes, peas, olives, parsley, and lemon juice and stir to combine. Serve hot.

Per serving: 438 calories, 9 g protein, 21 g fat (3 g sat), 55 g carbs, 735 mg sodium, 80 mg calcium, 7 g fiber

green gumbo

makes 4 servings

Green gumbo, also called gumbo z'herbes, is a hearty stew made with a generous amount of leafy greens, onion, celery, bell pepper, and jalapeño chiles. This variant features chewy spiced mushrooms instead of andouille sausage. Spoon-feed it to your sweetheart, buck naked or with cooked rice or other grains on top (or on the bottom—however you roll).

- ¼ cup whole wheat flour or unbleached all-purpose flour
- 2 tablespoons olive oil, or ¼ to ⅓ cup low-sodium vegetable broth
- 1 cup diced green bell pepper
- 1 cup diced celery
- 1 cup diced yellow onion
- 2 jalapeño chiles, seeded and finely diced
- 2 tablespoons minced garlic
- 20 leaves dark leafy greens (COLLARD GREENS, KALE, MUSTARD GREENS, SPINACH, SWISS CHARD, OR TURNIP GREENS, OR A COMBINATION), stemmed and cut into thin strips
- 3½ cups water
- 2 cups shredded green cabbage
- 1 bay leaf
- 6 ounces button or cremini mushrooms, coarsely chopped (ABOUT 3 CUPS)
- 1 tablespoon chili powder
- 1 teaspoon dried oregano
- 1 teaspoon dried thyme
- ¼ cup chopped fresh parsley, lightly packed
- 2 tablespoons nutritional yeast flakes
- Sea salt
- Freshly ground black pepper

1. Put the flour and 1½ tablespoons of the oil in a large soup pot and cook over medium heat, stirring occasionally, until golden brown, 10 to 12 minutes.

2. Add the bell pepper, celery, onion, chiles, and garlic and cook, stirring occasionally, until the vegetables are soft, 5 to 7 minutes.

3 Add the greens, water, cabbage, and bay leaf and stir to combine. Bring to a boil over high heat. Cover, decrease the heat to low, and simmer for 25 minutes.

4 While the gumbo is simmering, put the mushrooms and remaining ½ tablespoon of oil in a large cast-iron or nonstick skillet and cook over medium-high heat, stirring occasionally, until lightly browned, 7 to 8 minutes. Add the chili powder, oregano, and thyme and cook, stirring occasionally, for 2 minutes.

5 Add the mushrooms, parsley, and nutritional yeast to the gumbo and simmer, stirring occasionally, for 5 minutes. Remove and discard the bay leaf. Season with salt and pepper to taste. Serve hot.

Per serving: 206 calories, 9 g protein, 8 g fat (1 g sat), 29 g carbs, 92 mg sodium, 179 mg calcium, 7 g fiber
Note: Analysis doesn't include sea salt or freshly ground black pepper to taste.

pasta primavera

makes 4 servings

This light dish will ignite your passions. It's made with a colorful blend of pasta and springtime vegetables, all dressed in an entrancing sauce seasoned with white wine, lemon, vegan butter, and fresh herbs.

8 ounces small pasta (SUCH AS FARFALLE, PENNE, ROTINI, OR ZITI)
¾ cup low-sodium vegetable broth
1 large carrot, cut in half lengthwise and thinly sliced diagonally
1 cup asparagus, trimmed and thinly sliced diagonally into 1-inch pieces
1 cup diced orange or yellow bell pepper
2 cups coarsely chopped baby spinach or arugula, lightly packed
½ cup frozen peas or fava beans, thawed
½ cup thinly sliced green onions
¼ cup white wine (SUCH AS CHARDONNAY OR RIESLING)
¼ cup chopped fresh basil, lightly packed, or 2 tablespoons chopped fresh dill
¼ cup chopped fresh parsley, lightly packed
Zest and juice of 1 lemon (ABOUT 1 TABLESPOON ZEST AND ¼ CUP JUICE)
1½ tablespoons nutritional yeast flakes
1 tablespoon vegan butter
Sea salt
Freshly ground black pepper
Crushed red pepper flakes

1. To cook the pasta, fill a large saucepan two-thirds full with water and bring to a boil over medium-high heat. Add the pasta and cook, stirring occasionally, until tender. Drain in a colander.

2. While the pasta is boiling, cook the vegetables. Put ½ cup of the broth and the carrot, asparagus, and bell pepper in a large cast-iron or nonstick skillet. Cook over medium heat, stirring occasionally, for 5 minutes. Add the spinach, peas, and green onions and cook, stirring occasionally, until the vegetables are tender, 2 to 3 minutes.

3 Add the remaining ¼ cup of broth and the wine, basil, parsley, lemon zest and juice, nutritional yeast, and butter and cook, stirring occasionally, for 1 minute to blend the flavors. Remove from the heat.

4 Add the pasta and gently toss to combine. Season with salt, pepper, and red pepper flakes to taste. Serve hot.

turn-ons For a grain-free option, replace the pasta with 2 large zucchini that have been made into noodles with a spiralizer or vegetable peeler.

Per serving: 335 calories, 17 g protein, 5 g fat (1 g sat), 58 g carbs, 94 mg sodium, 59 mg calcium, 9 g fiber
Note: Analysis doesn't include sea salt, freshly ground black pepper, or crushed red pepper flakes to taste.

winter squash with apple-walnut stuffing

makes 4 servings

Getting stuffed can be a good thing, especially if you're a vegetable. Winter squash stuffed with bread cubes, apple, aromatic vegetables, dried fruit, and walnuts makes an outstanding dish during the colder months or as the centerpiece of any holiday or celebration meal.

- 2 medium winter squash (SUCH AS ACORN, CARNIVAL, DELICATA, OR SWEET DUMPLING)
- 4 cups whole-grain bread cubes
- 1 large apple, peeled and diced
- ½ cup diced red or yellow onion
- ½ cup diced celery
- 2 teaspoons olive oil, or ¼ cup low-sodium vegetable broth or water
- ⅓ cup coarsely chopped walnuts
- ¼ cup thinly sliced green onions
- ¼ cup dried cranberries or raisins
- 1½ tablespoons nutritional yeast flakes
- 1 teaspoon dried thyme
- ½ teaspoon ground cinnamon
- 1 cup low-sodium vegetable broth
- ¼ cup chopped fresh parsley, lightly packed
- Sea salt
- Freshly ground black pepper

1. Preheat the oven to 375 degrees F.

2. Cut the squash in half from the stem to the bottom. Using a spoon, scoop out the seeds and discard. Put the squash halves cut-side up in a 13 x 9-inch baking pan. Put about one inch of water in the bottom of the pan. Bake for 15 minutes.

3. While the squash is baking, make the stuffing. Put the bread cubes on a baking sheet and let sit for 15 minutes to dry out a little.

4 Put the apple, onion, celery, and oil in a large cast-iron or nonstick skillet and cook over medium heat, stirring occasionally, for 5 minutes. Add the walnuts, green onions, cranberries, nutritional yeast, thyme, and cinnamon and cook, stirring occasionally, for 3 minutes.

5 Transfer the bread cubes to a large bowl. Add the apple mixture, broth, and parsley and gently stir to moisten the bread cubes. Season with salt and pepper to taste.

6 Remove the squash from the oven. Fill the cavities evenly with the stuffing and bake for 15 to 20 minutes, until the squash is tender and the stuffing is lightly browned. Serve hot.

Per serving: 294 calories, 11 g protein, 10 g fat (1 g sat), 47 g carbs, 97 mg sodium, 139 mg calcium, 10 g fiber
Note: Analysis doesn't include sea salt or freshly ground black pepper to taste.

sweet-and-sour tofu and vegetables

makes 4 servings

The human tongue readily distinguishes between sweet and sour flavors. These contrasting tastes are often culinary mates because sometimes opposites really do attract. Dish up this saucy combination over hot rice or grains.

SWEET-AND-SOUR SAUCE

1 can (15 OUNCES) pineapple chunks
2 tablespoons ketchup
2 tablespoons reduced-sodium tamari or coconut aminos
2 tablespoons rice vinegar or cider vinegar
2 tablespoons light brown sugar or coconut sugar
1 tablespoon peeled and grated fresh ginger
1 tablespoon cornstarch

TOFU AND VEGGIES

8 ounces firm or extra-firm tofu
2 teaspoons cornstarch
1 tablespoon sunflower oil or other oil
1½ cups small broccoli florets
2 medium carrots, thinly sliced diagonally
2 large stalks celery, thinly sliced diagonally
1 medium orange or red bell pepper, cut into 1-inch pieces
½ medium green bell pepper, cut into 1-inch pieces
½ small red onion, cut into half moons

1. To make the sauce, drain the juice from the pineapple into a small bowl. Put the pineapple on a small plate and set aside. Add the ketchup, tamari, vinegar, brown sugar, ginger, and cornstarch to the pineapple juice and whisk to combine.

2. To prep the tofu, gently squeeze it over the sink to remove the excess water. Put the tofu in a colander in the sink, cover with a plate, put a heavy can (or other heavy object) on top of the plate, and let the tofu press for 20 minutes.

3. Cut the tofu into 1-inch cubes and put them on a large plate. Sprinkle the cornstarch over the top, then gently toss to evenly coat the cubes on all sides.

4 Put the tofu and oil in a large cast-iron or nonstick skillet and cook over medium heat, stirring occasionally, until lightly browned on all sides, 10 to 12 minutes. Transfer the tofu to a large plate using a slotted spoon.

5 Put the broccoli, carrots, celery, orange bell pepper, green bell pepper, and onion in the skillet and cook, stirring occasionally, until the vegetables are crisp-tender, 3 to 5 minutes. Add the reserved pineapple and cook, stirring occasionally, for 1 minute.

6 Add the reserved tofu cubes and sauce and cook, stirring constantly, until the sauce thickens, 1 to 2 minutes. Serve hot.

SWEET-AND-SOUR TEMPEH AND VEGETABLES: Replace the tofu with 1 package (8 ounces) tempeh, cut into 1-inch cubes. The tempeh doesn't need to be pressed.

Per serving: 268 calories, 11 g protein, 8 g fat (1 g sat), 44 g carbs, 483 mg sodium, 188 mg calcium, 6 g fiber

pesto-swirled polenta

makes 4 servings

Italians have a reputation for being amorous. Maybe that's due to their simple, come-hither foods that are irresistable yet comforting. Polenta is among them. If you've got cornmeal in your cupboard, you can quickly whip up this soft, satisfying dish. It's garnished with a decorative swirl of fresh pesto to tickle your fancy and have you (or your heartthrob) begging for more.

HERB PESTO

1½ cups fresh basil leaves, lightly packed
1 cup parsley leaves, lightly packed
¼ cup pine nuts, toasted, or ⅓ cup walnuts, toasted
2 tablespoons nutritional yeast flakes
1 tablespoon olive oil
1 tablespoon water
3 large cloves garlic
½ teaspoon sea salt
⅛ teaspoon ground black pepper

POLENTA

6 cups water
¾ teaspoon sea salt
½ teaspoon ground black pepper
1½ cups medium-grind or coarse cornmeal
2 tablespoons nutritional yeast flakes
1 tablespoon olive oil or vegan butter (OPTIONAL)
Crushed red pepper flakes (OPTIONAL)

1. To make the pesto, put all the ingredients in a food processor and process until smooth. Scrape down the container with a silicone spatula and process for 15 seconds longer.

2. To make the polenta, put the water, salt, and pepper in a large saucepan. Bring to a boil over high heat. Decrease the heat to medium. Slowly whisk in the cornmeal (to prevent lumps) and cook, whisking constantly, until the mixture begins to boil again, 1 to 2 minutes.

3 Decrease the heat to low. Cover and simmer, stirring every 10 minutes with a long-handled spoon, until the polenta is very thick and begins to pull away from the sides of the saucepan, 30 to 35 minutes. Remove from the heat.

4 Add the nutritional yeast and optional oil and stir to combine. Drop 2 tablespoons of the pesto over each serving, then snake a knife through the two mixtures to create a swirl effect. Garnish each serving with red pepper flakes if desired. Serve hot.

turn-ons For a heartier dish, top each serving with ⅓ cup of Lemon-Herb Roasted Chickpeas (page 146) or 1 Seitan Sausage (page 114), coarsely chopped.

Per serving: 747 calories, 21 g protein, 2 g fat (2 g sat), 136 g carbs, 660 mg sodium, 104 mg calcium, 16 g fiber

bacon mac-n-cheese

makes 4 servings

There's no denying the magnetism of comfort foods. This dish is so soothing, each forkful feels like a warm, lingering embrace.

CHEESY SAUCE

1½ cups water
1 medium carrot, diced
¼ cup raw cashews
¼ cup diced yellow onion
¼ cup diced orange or red bell pepper
2 large cloves garlic
3 tablespoons nutritional yeast flakes
2 teaspoons tapioca starch or cornstarch
1 teaspoon mellow or white miso
½ teaspoon chili powder
½ teaspoon smoked or sweet paprika
½ teaspoon sea salt
¼ teaspoon ground black pepper

MACARONI AND BACON

8 ounces elbow macaroni
Sea salt
Freshly ground black pepper
4 slices Tempeh Bacon (PAGE 116), coarsely chopped, or 1 recipe Coconut Bacon (PAGE 102)

1 To make the sauce, put the water, carrot, cashews, onion, bell pepper, and garlic in a medium saucepan and bring to a boil over high heat. Cover, decrease the heat to low, and cook until the vegetables are soft, 8 to 10 minutes. Remove from the heat. Let cool for 5 minutes.

2 Transfer to a blender. Add the nutritional yeast, tapioca starch, miso, chili powder, paprika, salt, and pepper and process until smooth. Scrape down the container with a silicone spatula and process for 15 seconds longer.

3 Pour the sauce into the medium saucepan and cook over medium heat, whisking occasionally, until very thick, 3 to 5 minutes. Remove from the heat.

4 To cook the macaroni, fill a large saucepan two-thirds full with water and bring to a boil over medium-high heat. Add the macaroni and cook, stirring occasionally, until tender. Drain in a colander and put it back in the large saucepan.

5 Add the sauce and stir to combine. Season with salt and pepper to taste. Scatter the tempeh bacon over the top or stir it in. Serve hot.

MUSHROOM MAC-N-CHEESE: Replace the tempeh bacon with 3 cups of thinly sliced button or cremini mushrooms. Cook the mushrooms in a skillet with ¼ cup of water or 1½ teaspoons of olive oil until tender, then stir into the finished mac-n-cheese.

Per serving: 598 calories, 26 g protein, 9 g fat (2 g sat), 102 g carbs, 531 mg sodium, 86 mg calcium, 7 g fiber
Note: Analysis doesn't include sea salt or freshly ground black pepper to taste.

BBQ seitan strips

makes 12 strips, 4 servings

For these vegan ribs, homemade seitan is patted into a baking pan, scored into strips, then partially baked. Next, the strips are covered with a sweet-and-spicy barbecue sauce and baked until lip-smacking good. Serve them as a main dish, or cut them into cubes and add them to bean or grain dishes.

SWEET-N-SPICY BBQ SAUCE

⅔ cup ketchup
2 tablespoons grated yellow onion
2 large cloves garlic, minced
1½ tablespoons cider vinegar
1½ tablespoons molasses or maple syrup, or 2 tablespoons coconut sugar
1 tablespoon bourbon (OPTIONAL)
1 tablespoon spicy brown or whole-grain mustard
1½ teaspoons chili powder
½ teaspoon ground cumin
½ teaspoon ground coriander
½ teaspoon sea salt
¼ teaspoon ground black pepper
¼ teaspoon liquid smoke (OPTIONAL)
⅛ teaspoon cayenne or hot sauce

SEITAN STRIPS

1 cup vital wheat gluten
¼ cup chickpea flour
2 tablespoons nutritional yeast flakes
1 teaspoon garlic powder
1 teaspoon onion powder
1 cup water
2 tablespoons tahini, peanut butter, or other nut or seed butter
1 tablespoon reduced-sodium tamari or coconut aminos

1 To make the sauce, put all the ingredients in a small saucepan and cook over low heat, stirring occasionally, until hot and bubbly, about 8 minutes. Remove from the heat.

2 Preheat the oven to 350 degrees F. Lightly oil a 9-inch square baking pan or mist it with cooking spray.

3 To make the seitan strips, put the vital wheat gluten, chickpea flour, nutritional yeast, garlic powder, and onion powder in a large bowl and stir to combine. Put the water, tahini, and tamari in a small bowl and stir to combine. Pour into the dry ingredients and stir to combine. Knead the mixture in the bowl until it forms a smooth and pliable dough, 1 to 2 minutes. Let rest for 5 minutes.

4 Transfer the dough to the prepared baking pan and flatten it with your hands to cover the bottom of the pan. Using a sharp knife, cut the dough lengthwise into six strips, give the pan a one-quarter turn, and cut the dough widthwise through the middle of each strip to yield twelve strips.

5 Bake for 25 minutes. Remove from the oven. Loosen the seitan from the sides and bottom of the pan with a metal spatula, then cut it into twelve strips again. Spread half the sauce over the strips. Bake for 7 minutes.

6 Remove from the oven. Carefully flip the strips over using a metal spatula. Spread the remaining sauce over the top. Bake for 8 to 10 minutes longer, until the strips are firm to the touch and the sauce is slightly caramelized. Let cool slightly before serving. Serve hot, room temperature, or cold.

Per serving: 276 calories, 13 g protein, 7 g fat (1 g sat), 45 g carbs, 921 mg sodium, 153 mg calcium, 5 g fiber

supper-sized stuffed florentine portobellos

makes 4 servings

Stuffed button mushrooms are typically served as an appetizer. Those bite-sized morsels were the inspiration for these supper-worthy stuffed portobellos. They feature a savory spinach-based filling that's topped with mozzarella cheese. One bite and your sweetie will be murmuring sweet nothings in your ear.

- ⅓ cup hot water
- 5 whole sun-dried tomatoes, or ⅓ cup chopped sun-dried tomatoes (NOT PACKED IN OIL)
- 4 large portobello mushrooms
- ½ cup finely diced celery
- ½ cup finely diced yellow onion
- ½ cup thinly sliced green onions
- 1 tablespoon olive oil
- 8 ounces firm or extra-firm tofu
- 1½ cups coarsely chopped baby spinach or arugula, lightly packed
- 1½ tablespoons minced garlic
- 1½ teaspoons dried basil
- 1½ teaspoons dried oregano
- ¾ cup dry bread crumbs or blanched almond flour
- 2 tablespoons nutritional yeast flakes
- 2 tablespoons chopped fresh parsley
- ½ teaspoon sea salt
- ½ teaspoon ground black pepper
- ¾ cup shredded vegan mozzarella cheese

1. Put the water and sun-dried tomatoes in a small bowl. Let sit for 10 minutes to rehydrate and soften the tomatoes. Drain. If using whole sun-dried tomatoes, coarsely chop them and set aside.
2. Preheat the oven to 375 degrees F. Line a baking sheet with parchment paper or a silicone baking mat.
3. Remove the stems from the mushrooms and finely chop them. Put the mushroom caps stem-side up on the lined baking sheet.

4 To make the filling, put the chopped mushroom stems, celery, onion, green onions, and oil in a large cast-iron or nonstick skillet and cook over medium-high heat, stirring occasionally, for 5 minutes. Crumble the tofu into the skillet and cook, stirring occasionally, for 3 minutes.

5 Add the reserved sun-dried tomatoes, spinach, garlic, basil, and oregano and cook, stirring occasionally, for 2 minutes. Remove from the heat. Add the bread crumbs, nutritional yeast, parsley, salt, and pepper and stir to combine.

6 Spoon the filling evenly into the mushroom caps. Sprinkle with the cheese. Bake for 22 to 25 minutes, until the mushrooms are tender. Serve hot.

Per serving: 217 calories, 12 g protein, 9 g fat (2 g sat), 26 g carbs, 521 mg sodium, 229 mg calcium, 5 g fiber

cornmeal-breaded tempeh

makes 8 pieces, 4 servings

Marinated tempeh is coated with a crunchy blend of cornmeal and pumpkin seeds, then baked until crisp and brown. Serve it as the main attraction with your favorites on the side—no one's counting, so invite as many sides as you like! The tempeh also makes an excellent sandwich filling or salad topper.

SEASONED BUTTERMILK AND TEMPEH

½ cup plain unsweetened soy milk or other nondairy milk
1 teaspoon reduced-sodium tamari
1 teaspoon cider vinegar or lemon juice
½ teaspoon garlic powder
½ teaspoon onion powder
2 packages (8 OUNCES EACH) tempeh

BREADING

½ cup raw pumpkin seeds
½ cup medium-grind cornmeal
3 tablespoons nutritional yeast flakes
2 teaspoons dried basil
1½ teaspoons chili powder
1 teaspoon dried oregano
¾ teaspoon ground coriander or cumin
½ teaspoon sea salt
¼ teaspoon ground black pepper

1. To make the seasoned buttermilk, put the soy milk, tamari, vinegar, garlic powder, and onion powder in a 13 x 9-inch baking pan and whisk to combine. Let sit for 5 minutes to thicken.
2. Cut each block of tempeh into four pieces. Pierce each piece several times along its length with a fork. Flip the tempeh over and pierce the other side in the same manner.
3. Put the tempeh in the buttermilk mixture and flip over each piece to evenly coat all sides. Let marinate in the refrigerator for at least 1 hour.

4 Preheat the oven to 400 degrees F. Line a baking sheet with parchment paper or a silicone baking mat.

5 To make the breading, put all the ingredients in a food processor and process until the pumpkin seeds are finely ground, 1 to 2 minutes. Transfer to a large plate.

6 Working with one piece at a time, put the tempeh in the breading, lightly pressing it down and flipping it over as needed to evenly coat all sides.

7 Arrange the breaded tempeh on the lined baking sheet, spacing the pieces two inches apart. Bake for 20 minutes. Remove from the oven and flip over each piece with a fork. Bake for 15 to 20 minutes longer, until the breading is lightly browned and crispy. Serve hot.

Per serving: 405 calories, 30 g protein, 22 g fat (4 g sat), 30 g carbs, 306 mg sodium, 208 mg calcium, 4 g fiber

coconut-crusted cutlets with sweet thai chili sauce

makes 8 cutlets, 4 servings

Pressing the tofu for this recipe takes twenty minutes, and marinating takes an hour, so summon your lover behind closed doors so you can work up an appetite while you wait! Serve this sensational tofu with the dipping sauce on the side, accompanied by stir-fried vegetables and rice to make a spectacular stay-at-home takeout meal.

TOFU AND MARINADE

1 pound firm or extra-firm tofu
3 tablespoons warm water
1 tablespoon ground flaxseeds or flaxseed meal
2 tablespoons reduced-sodium tamari
1 tablespoon minced garlic
1 tablespoon peeled and grated fresh ginger

SWEET THAI CHILI SAUCE

1 cup coconut water
½ cup unbleached cane sugar
⅓ cup rice vinegar or cider vinegar
1½ tablespoons minced garlic
1½ tablespoons peeled and grated fresh ginger
2 tablespoons cold water
1 tablespoon cornstarch
1½ teaspoons crushed red pepper flakes
1½ teaspoons hot sauce
Sea salt (OPTIONAL)

BREADING

⅔ cup unsweetened shredded dried coconut
⅓ cup blanched almond flour
2 tablespoons coconut sugar or unbleached cane sugar
½ teaspoon garlic powder
¼ teaspoon sea salt
¼ teaspoon ground black pepper

1. To prep the tofu, gently squeeze the block of tofu over the sink to remove excess water. Put the tofu in a colander in the sink, cover with a plate, put a heavy can (or other heavy object) on top of the plate, and let the tofu press for 20 minutes.

2 Cut the pressed tofu lengthwise into eight equal slices. Pierce each slice several times along its length with a fork. Flip each slice over and pierce the other side in the same manner.

3 To make the marinade, put the water and flaxseeds in a 9-inch square baking pan and whisk to combine. Let sit for 10 minutes to thicken into a gel.

4 Add the tamari, garlic, and ginger and whisk to combine. Add the tofu and flip over each slice to evenly coat all sides. Let marinate in the refrigerator for at least 1 hour.

5 To make the sauce, put the coconut water, sugar, vinegar, garlic, and ginger in a small saucepan and stir to combine. Bring to a boil over high heat. Decrease the heat to medium and cook, stirring occasionally, for 3 minutes.

6 Put the cold water and cornstarch in a small bowl and stir to combine. Add the cornstarch mixture, red pepper flakes, and hot sauce to the saucepan and cook, whisking occasionally, until the sauce thickens, 1 to 2 minutes. Remove from the heat and let cool slightly. Season with salt to taste if desired.

7 Preheat the oven to 400 degrees F. Line a baking sheet with parchment paper or a silicone baking mat.

8 To make the breading, put all the ingredients on a large plate and toss with your fingers to combine. Working with one slice at a time, put the tofu in the breading mixture, lightly pressing it down and flipping it over as needed to evenly coat all sides.

9 Arrange the breaded tofu in a single layer on the lined baking sheet, spacing the slices two inches apart. Bake for 25 minutes. Remove from the oven and flip over each slice with a fork. Bake for 15 to 20 minutes longer, until the breading is golden brown and crispy.

Per serving: 542 calories, 16 g protein, 32 g fat (22 g sat), 46 g carbs, 667 mg sodium, 214 mg calcium, 7 g fiber
Note: Analysis doesn't include sea salt to taste in the sauce.

hot-tamale pie

makes 4 servings

Can't resist hot and spicy? Then scratch that itch with this tempting hot-tamale pie. It features a chili filling with a cornbread topping. Consider your fantasies fulfilled!

CHILI FILLING

½ cup water

½ cup diced red or yellow onion

½ cup diced orange or red bell pepper

½ cup frozen corn kernels

½ cup peeled and diced sweet potato

½ cup diced zucchini

1 jalapeño chile, seeded and thinly sliced

1½ tablespoons minced garlic

2 teaspoons chili powder

1 teaspoon dried oregano

½ teaspoon ground cumin

½ teaspoon ground coriander

¼ teaspoon chipotle chile powder or cayenne

1 can (14 OUNCES) crushed tomatoes (FOR A SMOKY FLAVOR, USE FIRE-ROASTED TOMATOES WITH GREEN CHILES)

1 can (15 OUNCES) beans (SUCH AS BLACK BEANS, KIDNEY BEANS, PINTO BEANS, OR MIXED BEANS), drained and rinsed

¼ cup chopped fresh cilantro or parsley, lightly packed

Sea salt

Freshly ground black pepper

CORNBREAD TOPPING

⅔ cup medium-grind cornmeal

½ cup whole wheat pastry flour

2 teaspoons baking powder

¼ teaspoon sea salt

¾ cup plain unsweetened nondairy milk

1½ tablespoons sunflower oil or other oil

1 Preheat the oven to 400 degrees F. Lightly oil a 9-inch square or round baking pan or mist it with cooking spray.

2 To make the chili filling, put the water, onion, bell pepper, corn, sweet potato, zucchini, chile, and garlic in a large cast-iron or nonstick skillet and cook over medium heat, stirring occasionally, for 7 minutes. Add the chili powder, oregano, cumin, coriander, and chipotle chile powder and cook, stirring occasionally, until the vegetables are tender and the water has evaporated, 2 to 3 minutes. Remove from the heat.

3 Add the tomatoes, beans, and cilantro and stir to combine. Season with salt and pepper to taste. Transfer to the prepared baking pan.

4 To make the topping, put the cornmeal, flour, baking powder, and salt in a small bowl and whisk to combine. Add the milk and oil and whisk until smooth. Pour over the filling and smooth the top with a silicone spatula.

5 Bake for 20 to 25 minutes, until the topping is lightly browned. Let sit for 5 minutes before serving. Serve hot.

Per serving: 329 calories, 10 g protein, 7 g fat (1 g sat), 57 g carbs, 141 mg sodium, 205 mg calcium, 10 g fiber

Note: Analysis doesn't include sea salt or freshly ground black pepper to taste.

pasta puttanesca

makes 4 servings

Although the Italian word "puttanesca" roughly translates to "ladies of the night," the name was likely a nod to women who worked the night shift and needed to prepare a quick, tasty meal, not a reference to the sex trade. While there may always be some disagreement about the origin of the sauce, there's no dispute that its pungent aroma is a potent lure.

8 ounces spaghetti or linguine
⅔ cup diced yellow onion
⅔ cup diced red or green bell pepper
2 teaspoons olive oil, or ¼ cup low-sodium vegetable broth
2 tablespoons minced garlic
1 teaspoon dried oregano
½ teaspoon crushed red pepper flakes
1 can (14 OUNCES) **crushed tomatoes** (FOR A SMOKY FLAVOR, USE FIRE-ROASTED TOMATOES)
½ cup pitted kalamata or black olives, sliced
2 tablespoons capers
1 tablespoon nutritional yeast flakes, plus more for garnish
⅓ cup chopped fresh basil, lightly packed
3 tablespoons chopped fresh parsley, lightly packed
Sea salt
Freshly ground black pepper

1. To cook the spaghetti, fill a large saucepan two-thirds full with water and bring to a boil over medium-high heat. Add the spaghetti and cook, stirring occasionally, until tender. Reserve ¼ cup of the cooking water. Drain the spaghetti in a colander.
2. While the spaghetti is cooking, make the sauce. Put the onion, bell pepper, and oil in a large cast-iron or nonstick skillet and cook over medium heat, stirring occasionally, for 5 minutes. Add the garlic, oregano, and red pepper flakes, and cook, stirring occasionally, until the vegetables are tender, 2 to 3 minutes.
3. Add the reserved cooking water, tomatoes, olives, capers, and nutritional yeast and cook, stirring occasionally, for 2 minutes. Add the basil and parsley and cook for 1 minute to blend the flavors. Remove from the heat. Season with salt and pepper to taste.
4. Add the spaghetti and gently toss to coat with the sauce. Serve hot, garnished with additional nutritional yeast.

Per serving: 305 calories, 11 g protein, 6 g fat (1 g sat), 53 g carbs, 384 mg sodium, 72 mg calcium, 6 g fiber
Note: Analysis doesn't include sea salt or freshly ground black pepper to taste.

mushroom and veggie fajitas

makes 4 servings

Fajitas are a Tex-Mex specialty, and this fabulous vegan version checks all the right boxes. Mushrooms, onions, and bell peppers are marinated in a zesty lime dressing, then cooked and folded in flour tortillas along with avocado and tomatoes.

Zest and juice of 2 limes (ABOUT 4 TEASPOONS ZEST AND ¼ CUP JUICE)

2 tablespoons minced garlic

1½ tablespoons olive oil

1 teaspoon dried oregano

1 teaspoon chili powder, or ½ teaspoon chipotle chile powder and ¼ teaspoon crushed red pepper flakes

2 portobello mushrooms, halved and cut into ½-inch-thick slices, or 2½ cups sliced button or cremini mushrooms

1 large red or yellow onion, cut into ½-inch-thick slices

1 medium green bell pepper, cut into ½-inch-thick slices

1 medium orange or red bell pepper, cut into ½-inch-thick slices

1 jalapeño chile, seeded and finely diced (OPTIONAL)

⅓ cup chopped fresh cilantro, lightly packed

Sea salt

Freshly ground black pepper

4 (8-INCH OR LARGER) **flour tortillas**

1 avocado, thinly sliced

1 cup diced tomatoes

1 Put the lime zest and juice, garlic, oil, oregano, and chili powder in a large bowl and stir to combine.

2 Add the mushrooms, onion, green bell pepper, orange bell pepper, optional chile, and cilantro and stir to combine. Season with salt and pepper to taste. Let marinate for 10 minutes.

3 Transfer the mushroom mixture to a large cast-iron or nonstick skillet and cook over medium-high heat, stirring occasionally, until the vegetables are tender, 8 to 10 minutes

4 To assemble the fajitas, put each tortilla on a large plate. Divide the vegetable mixture equally among them, arranging it horizontally in the center of the tortillas. Top with the avocado and tomatoes. Serve hot.

Per serving: 238 calories, 5 g protein, 16 g fat (3 g sat), 23 g carbs, 26 mg sodium, 50 mg calcium, 7 g fiber
Note: Analysis doesn't include sea salt or freshly ground black pepper to taste.

happy endings

Everyone loves a happy ending, whether it's the completion of a sappy story or the climax of a sizzling sexcapade. In this section you'll discover all you need to satisfy your sweet tooth and achieve that satisfying finish.

raw fruity delight

makes 2 servings

Fresh fruit is most seductive when preparation is minimal and presentation is simple. After all, when you're naturally sweet and juicy, you don't need to hide behind anything elaborate. Spoon or slurp this luscious purée, and don't forget to lick the bowl so you don't miss a single drop.

¼ cup orange juice

4 pitted soft dates

2 nectarines or peaches, peeled and diced

1 mango, peeled, pitted, and diced

¾ cup whole berries (SUCH AS BLUEBERRIES, BLACKBERRIES, OR RASPBERRIES), or ⅔ cup sliced strawberries

1 kiwi, peeled, quartered lengthwise, and thinly sliced

¼ cup pomegranate seeds, or 2 tablespoons dried goji berries

1. Put the juice and dates in a small bowl. Let sit for 15 minutes to plump the dates.
2. Transfer the juice and dates to a food processor and process for 30 seconds. Scrape down the container with a silicone spatula. Add the nectarines and mango and process until smooth.
3. Pour into a medium bowl. Scatter the berries, kiwi, and pomegranate seeds over the top. Serve immediately.

Per serving: 328 calories, 5 g protein, 2 g fat (0.2 g sat), 81 g carbs, 4 mg sodium, 47 mg calcium, 9 g fiber

pop-your-cherry pudding

makes 2 servings

This no-cook pudding contains energy-enhancing chia seeds that thicken without heat. The cherries, almonds, coconut milk, and maca powder create quite a compelling combination. This tasty treat makes an exquisite breakfast, dessert, or snack. You'll be instantly smitten.

1½ cups fresh or frozen pitted cherries
1 cup plain or vanilla coconut milk beverage
6 tablespoons sliced raw almonds
2 tablespoons agave nectar, maple syrup, or coconut sugar
2 teaspoons maca powder
1 teaspoon vanilla extract
½ teaspoon almond extract, or 2 tablespoons amaretto
3 tablespoons chia seeds

1. Coarsely chop ½ cup of the cherries. Transfer them to a small bowl and refrigerate.
2. Put the remaining cup of cherries, the milk, 4 tablespoons of the almonds, and the agave nectar, maca powder, vanilla extract, and almond extract in a blender and process until smooth. Scrape down the container with a silicone spatula. Add the chia seeds and process for 15 seconds.
3. Transfer to a small bowl and refrigerate until the chia seeds swell and thicken the mixture into a pudding, about 1 hour.
4. Before serving, whisk the mixture to break up any clumps of chia seeds. Top each serving with the reserved cherries and almonds.

RIPE-AND-READY RASPBERRY PUDDING: Replace the cherries with 1½ cups of fresh or frozen raspberries. Omit the almond extract.

Per serving: 354 calories, 10 g protein, 18 g fat (1 g sat), 50 g carbs, 75 mg sodium, 393 mg calcium, 14 g fiber

spiked dark chocolate truffles

makes 12 truffles, 4 servings

Transform store-bought dark chocolate into vegan truffles with very little effort. These spirited rascals will literally melt in your mouth.

TRUFFLES

2 bars (3 OUNCES EACH) vegan dark chocolate, coarsely chopped, or 1 cup vegan chocolate chips

¼ cup full-fat coconut milk

2 tablespoons coconut oil

2 tablespoons red wine, or 1 tablespoon amaretto, coffee liqueur, rum, whiskey, or other liquor or liqueur

½ teaspoon vanilla extract

Pinch sea salt

Cacao powder or unsweetened cocoa powder

COATING OPTIONS

Additional cacao powder or unsweetened cocoa powder

Cacao nibs

Finely ground nuts

Powdered sugar

Unsweetened shredded dried coconut

1. Put the chocolate, coconut milk, coconut oil, wine, vanilla extract, and salt in a small bowl and microwave for 1 to 2 minutes to melt the chocolate. Alternatively, put the chocolate in a double boiler over medium-low heat until the chocolate is melted.

2. Transfer the chocolate mixture to an 8-inch square baking pan. Refrigerate until firm but pliable, about 1 hour.

3. Line a large plate with parchment or waxed paper. Portion the chocolate mixture using 1 tablespoonful for each truffle and immediately put on the plate. Lightly coat your hands with cacao powder, roll each portion into a ball, then put the truffles back on the plate. Refrigerate for 30 minutes.

4. Line another large plate with parchment or waxed paper. Roll each truffle in the toppings of your choice, then put them on the lined plate. Refrigerate the truffles for 15 minutes before serving. Store in an airtight container in the refrigerator.

Per serving: 327 calories, 4 g protein, 23 g fat (18 g sat), 26 g carbs, 95 mg sodium, 83 mg calcium, 2 g fiber
Note: Analysis doesn't include coating options.

turn-ons Get a little kinky! Vary the flavor of the truffles by adding ¼ teaspoon of ground spices (such as cardamom, cayenne, or cinnamon) or flavoring extract (such as almond, coconut, or peppermint) to the melted chocolate mixture.

after-dark chocolate sauce and fondue

makes 1⅔ cups

You can make this rich, velvety sauce a bit boozy or a smidge spicy, whichever suits your mood. It makes a delectable topping for desserts and nondairy ice cream, or you can let it firm up in the fridge and use it as body paint for your sweetheart. It also makes a romantic fondue for two.

1¼ cups plain or vanilla soy milk or other nondairy milk

¼ cup cacao powder or unsweetened cocoa powder

2 tablespoons agave nectar, maple syrup, or unbleached cane sugar

Pinch sea salt

1 cup vegan chocolate chips, or 2 bars (3 OUNCES EACH) **vegan dark chocolate, coarsely chopped**

1½ teaspoons vanilla extract

1 tablespoon liqueur (SUCH AS CHERRY, COFFEE, OR ORANGE)**, bourbon, or rum** (OPTIONAL)

¼ teaspoon ground cinnamon or cayenne (OPTIONAL)

1 Put the milk, cacao powder, agave nectar, and salt in a small saucepan and whisk to combine. Cook over medium heat, whisking occasionally, until the mixture just begins to boil, 2 to 3 minutes.

2 Remove from the heat. Add the chocolate chips and vanilla extract and whisk until the chocolate is completely melted. Whisk in the optional liqueur and cinnamon. Serve hot, warm, or room temperature. Store leftovers in an airtight container in the refrigerator. Chilling the sauce will thicken it to the consistency of ganache.

FONDUE FOR TWO: Serve the warm sauce with your favorite dippers: whole strawberries or raspberries, whole cherries, whole seedless grapes, thick banana slices, pineapple chunks, pretzels, or large cubes of cake. Dipping fingers and toes is optional.

Per ⅓ cup: 221 calories, 4 g protein, 11 g fat (7 g sat), 29 g carbs, 112 mg sodium, 182 mg calcium, 3 g fiber

filled figs your way

makes 12 figs, 4 servings

To appreciate a fig's inner beauty, split it at the top, then gently pull it open to reveal its succulent interior. Although you could savor it in its birthday suit, why not embellish it with something scrumptious? Three filling choices are presented for your perusal because sometimes you just need a few racy options.

FIGS

12 fresh figs

FILLINGS (CHOOSE ONE)

Mock Marzipan Filling

1¼ cups sliced raw almonds

¾ cup powdered sugar

1 tablespoon agave nectar

1 tablespoon water

¾ teaspoon vanilla extract

¼ teaspoon almond extract

Strawberry Cream Cheese and Pistachio Filling

¾ cup Strawberry-Cashew Cream Cheese Spread (PAGE 104)

2 to 3 tablespoons finely chopped raw or roasted pistachios

Coconut Cream Filling

¾ cup Whipped Coconut Cream (PAGE 215)

3 tablespoons unsweetened shredded dried coconut, raw or lightly toasted

1 To prep each fig, cut off the stem and discard. Cut an X into the fig (from the stem toward the bottom) without cutting all the way through, then gently open the top portion of the fig (like a budding flower). Put the figs on a large plate or platter and fill as desired.

2 **To make the marzipan filling,** reserve 12 of the sliced almonds for the garnish. Put the remaining almonds and the powdered sugar, agave nectar, water, vanilla extract, and almond extract in a food processor and process into a smooth paste. Transfer to a small bowl and refrigerate for 15 minutes. Roll 1 tablespoon of the filling into a log and put it into the center of a fig. Continue this process until all the filling is used up and all the figs are filled. Stick one of the reserved almonds into the center of each log as a garnish.

To make the strawberry cream cheese filling, put the spread in a pastry bag fitted with a star tip. Alternatively, put the spread in a small ziplock bag, seal the bag, then snip off one of the bottom corners with scissors. Decoratively pipe 1 tablespoon of the mixture in the center of each fig. Garnish with the pistachios.

To make the coconut cream filling, put the whipped coconut cream in a pastry bag fitted with a star tip. Alternatively, put the cream in a small ziplock bag, seal the bag, then snip off one of the bottom corners with scissors. Decoratively pipe 1 tablespoon of the cream in the center of each fig. Garnish with the coconut.

turn-ons When fresh figs aren't available, use dried figs or pitted medjool dates, cut in half lengthwise. Use half the amount of filling to sandwich the two halves together.

Per serving with Mock Marzipan Filling: 419 calories, 8 g protein, 15 g fat (1 g sat), 69 g carbs, 6 mg sodium, 173 mg calcium 19 g fiber

Per serving with Strawberry Cream Cheese and Pistachio Filling: 241 calories, 3 g protein, 7 g fat (0.4 g sat), 45 g carbs, 33 mg sodium, 101 mg calcium, 6 g fiber

Per serving with Coconut Cream Filling: 529 calories, 5 g protein, 37 g fat (30 g sat), 48 g carbs, 56 mg sodium, 92 mg calcium, 6 g fiber

vanilla-infused banana ice cream and partners

makes 2 servings

It's a breeze to make homemade ice cream with just a few vegan staples. Enjoy this soft serve straight up or all decked out. For an over-the-top sundae, fancy it up with chopped fruit and nuts, After-Dark Chocolate Sauce (page 203), and Whipped Coconut Cream (page 215). Like variety? We've got you covered with a slew of options.

2 large, very ripe bananas, broken into pieces and frozen

¼ cup plain or vanilla coconut milk beverage or other nondairy milk

1½ teaspoons vanilla extract

Put all the ingredients in a food processor or a blender with a tamper and process until smooth. Scrape down the container with a silicone spatula and process for 15 seconds longer. Serve immediately.

BERRY AND BANANA ICE CREAM: Add 1 cup of fresh blueberries, raspberries, or sliced strawberries, or 1 cup of frozen berries (do not thaw).

CHOCOLATE, PEANUT BUTTER, AND BANANA ICE CREAM: Decrease the milk to 2½ tablespoons. Add 3 tablespoons of peanut butter and 3 tablespoons of cacao powder or unsweetened cocoa powder.

MAPLE-WALNUT BANANA ICE CREAM: Replace the coconut milk with 2½ tablespoons of almond milk and 1½ tablespoons of maple syrup. Stir ⅓ cup of walnuts, toasted and coarsely chopped, into the finished ice cream.

PINEAPPLE AND BANANA SHERBET: Omit the vanilla extract. Add 1 cup of canned or frozen pineapple chunks.

Per serving: 131 calories, 2 g protein, 1 g fat (1 g sat), 32 g carbs, 3 mg sodium, 19 mg calcium, 4 g fiber
Note: Analysis does not include the partners.

cherries jubilee

makes 2 cups, 4 servings

Flambéed desserts make a dramatic presentation—just be sure to first check out the safety tips that follow. This showstopper is made by gently cooking cherries in a lemon-flavored syrup, dousing them with spirits, and setting them aflame. Serve them over nondairy ice cream, cake, or other desserts, or simply spoon them into your (or your sugar pie's) mouth.

1 pound fresh or frozen pitted cherries

⅓ cup unbleached cane sugar

2 tablespoons vegan butter

Zest and juice of ½ lemon (ABOUT 1½ TEASPOONS ZEST AND 2 TABLESPOONS JUICE)

¼ cup liqueur (SUCH AS AMARETTO, KIRSCH, OR ORANGE LIQUEUR) **or brandy**

1. Put the cherries and sugar in a large cast-iron or nonstick skillet and cook over medium-high heat, stirring occasionally, until the sugar is fully dissolved and the cherries are soft, 5 to 7 minutes.

2. Add the butter and lemon zest and juice and cook, stirring constantly, until the butter is melted, about 1 minute.

3. Using a long-handled metal spoon, stir in the liqueur. Carefully light a long match and hold it to the cherry mixture to ignite the alcohol (for a more dramatic effect, do this with the lights dimmed). When the flame has subsided and is small and blue, gently stir the mixture to cook off any remaining alcohol. Remove from the heat. Serve hot or warm.

SAFETY TIPS: When preparing any flambéed dish, be very careful to avoid getting burned or causing a fire. Don't wear long or hanging sleeves, and if you're wearing a tie, tuck it in. Keep hair pulled or tied back and away from the flame. After you ignite the alcohol, wait for the big flame to die down to a small blue flame before stirring the dish with a metal spoon to cook off any residual alcohol. This cooking method helps to reduce the strong flavor of the alcohol and caramelizes the sugars in the food. It also makes an entertaining presentation. Just in case anything goes awry, keep an appropriate-sized lid nearby to quickly snuff out the flames, and keep your fire extinguisher handy.

Per serving: 257 calories, 1 g protein, 6 g fat (2 g sat), 48 g carbs, 80 mg sodium, 12 mg calcium, 1 g fiber

mulled wine poached pears

makes 4 servings

Need to cuddle up with something warm and sweet on a chilly evening? This dessert is just the ticket. Its elegance belies its ease of preparation, so it's ideal to serve to that special someone you want to impress.

- **½ large orange**
- **2 cups red wine**
- **¼ cup maple syrup or light brown sugar**
- **1** (3-INCH) **cinnamon stick**
- **3 whole allspice berries, or ¼ teaspoon ground allspice**
- **3 whole cloves**
- **4 large pears**
- **Vanilla nondairy yogurt** (OPTIONAL)

1. Using a vegetable peeler, remove two or three long strips of the zest from the orange half and put them in a large saucepan. Add the wine, maple syrup, cinnamon stick, allspice, and cloves. Bring to a boil over high heat. Cover, decrease the heat to low, and simmer for 5 minutes.

2. While the wine mixture is cooking, peel the pears but leave the stems intact. Put the pears in the wine mixture and tilt them on their sides to submerge them as much as possible. Cover and cook until the pears are tender and easily pierced with the tip of a sharp knife, 15 to 20 minutes, turning the pears over every 5 minutes to ensure even coloring and cooking.

3. Remove from the heat and uncover the saucepan. Let the pears cool in the poaching liquid for 15 minutes. Using a slotted spoon, transfer the pears to a large plate or platter and set aside. Remove the orange peel, cinnamon stick, allspice, and cloves with the slotted spoon and discard them.

4. Bring the poaching liquid to a boil over medium heat. Cook until the liquid is reduced by half and thickens into a syrup, 10 to 15 minutes.

5. Serve the pears room temperature, drizzled with the reduced poaching liquid and topped with dollops of yogurt if desired.

Per serving: 286 calories, 1 g protein, 1 g fat (0.1 g sat), 52 g carbs, 14 mg sodium, 61 mg calcium, 8 g fiber

sugar-n-spice cookies

makes 30 cookies

The scent of cinnamon can be a potent aphrodisiac. If you're smitten by this fragrant spice, the aroma of these divine confections will curl your toes. The cookies are so tender they will melt in your or your sugar cookie's mouth.

2½ tablespoons water
1 teaspoon chia seeds
⅔ cup plus 2 tablespoons unbleached cane sugar
2 teaspoons ground cinnamon
3 cups blanched almond flour
¾ teaspoon baking soda
¼ teaspoon sea salt
4 tablespoons coconut oil, melted
1½ tablespoons vanilla extract

1. Preheat the oven to 350 degrees F. Line two baking sheets with parchment paper or silicone baking mats.
2. Put the water and chia seeds in a small bowl and stir to combine. Let sit for 10 minutes to thicken into a gel.
3. Put 2 tablespoons of the sugar and the cinnamon in a small bowl and stir to combine.
4. Put the remaining ⅔ cup of sugar and the almond flour, baking soda, and salt in a large bowl and stir to combine. Add the chia seed mixture, coconut oil, and vanilla extract and use a fork to work them into the flour mixture to form a soft dough.
5. Roll the dough into one-inch balls, then roll each ball in the cinnamon-sugar mixture to evenly coat all sides. Arrange the balls two inches apart on the lined baking sheets. Using a measuring cup or glass, slightly flatten each ball.
6. Bake for 10 to 12 minutes, until the cookies are set on top and lightly browned on the bottom and around the edges. Let cool completely on the baking sheets. Store in an airtight container at room temperature.

PINE NUT SUGAR COOKIES: Stir ½ cup of pine nuts, toasted, and 1 teaspoon of ground fennel into the finished cookie dough. Shape the dough into one-inch balls and roll them in unbleached cane sugar (don't add the cinnamon).

Per cookie: 106 calories, 3 g protein, 7 g fat (2 g sat), 8 g carbs, 53 mg sodium, 5 mg calcium, 1 g fiber

making whoopie pies

makes 12 sandwich cookies

In case you haven't heard of whoopie pies, they're just about the yummiest sandwich cookies ever. Here's the 411: Cakey dark-chocolate cookies are sandwiched together with a creamy buttercream frosting. Got it? Now let's make some whoopie!

COOKIES

1 cup whole wheat pastry flour
6 tablespoons cacao powder or unsweetened cocoa powder
½ teaspoon baking soda
¼ teaspoon baking powder
¼ teaspoon sea salt
½ cup light brown sugar, lightly packed
¼ cup vegan butter
¼ cup plain or vanilla nondairy yogurt
¼ cup plain or chocolate nondairy milk
½ teaspoon vanilla extract

BUTTERCREAM FROSTING

1¼ cups powdered sugar
2½ tablespoons vegan butter
1 tablespoon plain nondairy milk
1 teaspoon vanilla extract

1. Preheat the oven to 350 degrees F. Line two baking sheets with parchment paper or silicone baking mats.
2. To make the cookies, put the flour, cacao powder, baking soda, baking powder, and salt in a medium bowl and whisk to combine.
3. Put the brown sugar, butter, yogurt, milk, and vanilla extract in the bowl of an electric mixer and beat for 1 minute. Add the flour mixture and beat to form a thick batter, about 1 minute.
4. Portion the batter onto the lined baking sheets using 1 level tablespoon per cookie, spacing them two inches apart (twelve cookies per baking sheet). Slightly flatten each portion with your fingers.
5. Bake for 10 minutes, until the cookies are set on top (they will be soft). Let cool completely on the baking sheets.

6 While the cookies are cooling, make the buttercream frosting. Put all the ingredients in the bowl of an electric mixer and beat until light and fluffy, 2 to 3 minutes.

7 To assemble each whoopie pie, put 1 tablespoon of the buttercream frosting on the bottom of one cookie. Put another cookie (bottom-side in) on top and gently press the cookies together. Repeat with the remaining cookies and frosting. Store in an airtight container in the refrigerator.

Per sandwich cookie: 174 calories, 2 g protein, 7 g fat (2 g sat), 28 g carbs, 163 mg sodium, 35 mg calcium, 2 g fiber

amazing avocado-chocolate mousse

makes 2 servings

Avocado, banana, and chocolate might seem like strange bedfellows, but as with any threesome, each brings something unique and delightful to the relationship. Feel like playing dress-up? Adorn this lavish mousse with berries, cacao nibs, chopped chocolate, or—what else?—vegan whipped cream, of course! (Check out Whipped Coconut Cream, page 215).

1 banana, broken into pieces

1 avocado, diced

¼ cup almond butter, peanut butter, or other nut or seed butter

¼ cup cacao powder or unsweetened cocoa powder

2 teaspoons maca powder (OPTIONAL)

1 teaspoon vanilla extract

Pinch sea salt

1 Put all the ingredients in a food processor and process until smooth. Scrape down the container with a silicone spatula and process for 15 seconds longer.

2 Serve immediately or refrigerate before serving.

Per serving: 300 calories, 5 g protein, 22 g fat (5 g sat), 29 g carbs, 126 mg sodium, 30 mg calcium, 12 g fiber

vegan berry cheesecake

makes 8 servings

"Cheesecake" used to refer to photography, art, or films that portray women in stereotypical sexual attractiveness. While that's fine if that's your thing (no judging!), we'd rather take a bite of this rich, creamy dessert, dripping with juicy berries on top.

CRUST

1½ cups blanched almond flour

¼ cup light brown sugar, lightly packed

2 tablespoons vegan butter

FILLING

1 package (12 OUNCES) **extra-firm silken tofu**

2 packages (8 OUNCES EACH) **vegan cream cheese**

⅔ cup unbleached cane sugar

¼ cup cornstarch

Zest and juice of 1 lemon (ABOUT 1 TABLESPOON ZEST AND ¼ CUP JUICE)

1½ tablespoons vanilla extract

TOPPING

1 pint fresh berries (SUCH AS BLACKBERRIES, BLUEBERRIES, RASPBERRIES, OR SLICED STRAWBERRIES)

2 tablespoons unbleached cane sugar

4 tablespoons water

1½ teaspoons cornstarch

1. Preheat the oven to 350 degrees F. Lightly oil an 8-inch springform pan or mist it with cooking spray.
2. To make the crust, put all the ingredients in a food processor and process for 1 minute. Transfer to the prepared springform pan. Using your hands, evenly flatten the mixture to cover the bottom of the pan. Bake for 8 minutes. Remove from the oven. Let cool for 5 minutes.
3. To make the filling, put all the ingredients in a food processor and process until smooth. Scrape down the container with a silicone spatula and process for 15 seconds longer. Transfer to the crust and smooth the top with the silicone spatula.

4 Put the cheesecake on a baking sheet. Bake for 45 to 50 minutes, until the filling is set. Let cool for 30 minutes. Loosen the sides of the cheesecake from the pan with a knife. Chill in the refrigerator for at least 2 hours.

5 To make the topping, put the berries, sugar, and 2 tablespoons of the water in a small saucepan. Cook over medium heat, stirring occasionally, for 3 minutes. Put the remaining 2 tablespoons of water and the cornstarch in a small bowl and whisk to combine. Add the cornstarch mixture to the saucepan and cook, whisking occasionally, until the topping thickens, 1 to 2 minutes. Remove from the heat. Let cool for 10 minutes. Spoon the topping mixture over the cheesecake and refrigerate.

6 Before serving, loosen the sides of the cheesecake from the pan with a knife, and remove the outer ring of the springform pan. Dip a sharp knife in warm water and wipe on a paper towel before slicing the cheesecake. Store the cheesecake covered in the refrigerator.

Per serving: 396 calories, 15 g protein, 19 g fat (3 g sat), 42 g carbs, 288 mg sodium, 79 mg calcium, 6 g fiber

vanilla pound cake

makes 8 slices

Do "sweet, moist, and tender" turn you on? Then you'll fall in love with this pound cake. It has a moist, tender crumb, is dense (but not stupid), and is brimming with beguiling vanilla. Want to snazz it up a bit? Dust it with powdered sugar, serve it with a side of fresh berries, or top it with Cherries Jubilee (page 207). Is your heart pounding yet?

1⅔ cups unbleached all-purpose flour or whole wheat pastry flour
⅔ cup unbleached cane sugar
1 teaspoon baking soda
¼ teaspoon baking powder
¼ teaspoon sea salt
¾ cup vanilla nondairy milk
1 container (6 OUNCES) **vanilla nondairy yogurt**
1 tablespoon sunflower oil or other oil
1 tablespoon vanilla extract

1. Preheat the oven to 350 degrees F. Lightly oil an 8 x 4 x 2½-inch loaf pan or mist it with cooking spray.
2. Put the flour, sugar, baking soda, baking powder, and salt in a large bowl and whisk to combine.
3. Put the milk, yogurt, oil, and vanilla extract in a small bowl and whisk to combine. Add the milk mixture to the flour mixture and whisk to combine.
4. Transfer to the prepared loaf pan and smooth the top with a silicone spatula.
5. Bake for 30 to 35 minutes, until a toothpick inserted in the center comes out clean. Let cool in the pan for 5 minutes.
6. Loosen the sides of the cake from the pan with a knife. Invert the pan onto a rack and let the cake release naturally from the pan. Serve warm or room temperature. Store in an airtight container at room temperature.

GLUTEN-FREE VANILLA POUND CAKE: Replace the unbleached all-purpose flour with 1⅔ cups of gluten-free baking mix plus ½ teaspoon of xanthan gum.

LEMON–POPPY SEED POUND CAKE: Replace ¼ cup of the nondairy milk with the zest and juice of 1 lemon (about 1 tablespoon zest and ¼ cup juice). Stir 1½ tablespoons of poppy seeds into the finished cake batter.

VANILLA-BERRY POUND CAKE: Stir ½ cup of fresh or frozen berries (such as blackberries, blueberries, or red raspberries) into the finished cake batter.

Per serving: 408 calories, 10 g protein, 5 g fat (0.3 g sat), 80 g carbs, 248 mg sodium, 171 mg calcium, 4 g fiber

whipped coconut cream

makes 1½ cups

Chilling full-fat canned coconut milk causes the thick cream to rise to the top, separating it from the coconut water on the bottom. The cream can then be scooped out and blended to create a rich, fluffy topping. Dollop it on fresh berries, a special dessert, or your dear one, if you're feeling risqué!

2 cans (14 OUNCES EACH) **full-fat coconut milk, refrigerated for 8 to 12 hours**

⅓ cup powdered sugar

1½ teaspoons vanilla extract

1. Chill a large bowl and electric beaters in the freezer for 20 minutes.
2. Carefully open the cold coconut milk. Using a spoon, skim only the thick coconut cream from the top of each can, carefully avoiding the watery liquid in the bottom of the can. Put the coconut cream in the chilled bowl. (Use the remaining liquid for smoothies or discard it.)
3. Beat the coconut cream with an electric mixer until soft peaks form, 2 to 3 minutes.
4. Add the powdered sugar and vanilla extract and beat for 1 minute. Store in an airtight container in the refrigerator.

turn-ons For even easier preparation, replace the coconut milk with 1 can (14 ounces) of coconut cream, refrigerated for 8 to 12 hours. Coconut cream is usually located near the canned coconut milk in most grocery stores.

Per ¼ cup: 516 calories, 5 g protein, 49 g fat (39 g sat), 16 g carbs, 67 mg sodium, 0 mg calcium, 0 g fiber

devil's food cake with after-dark ganache

makes 8 slices

This dark-chocolate cake is devilishly good, but since it contains no oil, it's surprisingly guilt-free too. Through culinary alchemy, healthy ingredients are combined to provide sweetness and moisture without the need for added fat. The finished cake is glazed with a layer of dark-chocolate sauce, then briefly chilled to harden the sauce into a ganache.

1¼ cups cold coffee
1 large apple, peeled and diced
8 pitted soft dates (PREFERABLY MEDJOOL)
8 pitted prunes
⅔ cup cacao powder or unsweetened cocoa powder
⅔ cup light brown sugar or coconut sugar
1⅓ cups whole wheat pastry flour
1 teaspoon baking soda
½ teaspoon baking powder
½ teaspoon sea salt
½ teaspoon ground cinnamon
1 cup After-Dark Chocolate Sauce (PAGE 203)**, warm**

1 Preheat the oven to 350 degrees F. Lightly oil an 8-inch springform pan or 8-inch round cake pan or mist it with cooking spray.

2 Put the coffee, apple, dates, prunes, cacao powder, and brown sugar in a medium saucepan and stir thoroughly to combine. Partially cover and cook over medium heat, stirring occasionally, until the apple is soft, 5 to 7 minutes. Remove from the heat. Let cool for 5 minutes.

3 Transfer to a food processor and process until smooth. Scrape down the container with a silicone spatula. Add the flour, baking soda, baking powder, salt, and cinnamon and process until smooth. Scrape down the container with the silicone spatula and process for 15 seconds longer.

4 Pour into the prepared pan and smooth the top with the back of the silicone spatula.

5 Bake for 30 to 35 minutes, until a toothpick inserted in the center comes out clean. Let cool in the pan for 5 minutes.

6 Loosen the sides of the cake from the pan with a knife. If using a springform pan, remove the outer ring. If using a cake pan, invert the pan onto a rack and let the cake release naturally from the pan. Let cool completely.

7 Put the cooled cake on a plate. Slowly and evenly drizzle the warm chocolate sauce over the top of the cake, using a silicone spatula as needed to help cover the sides of the cake with the sauce. Put the cake in the refrigerator until the sauce hardens into a ganache, 10 to 15 minutes.

8 Let the cake sit at room temperature for 3 minutes before cutting. Dip a sharp knife in warm water and wipe on a paper towel before slicing. Store the cake covered in the refrigerator.

Per serving: 591 calories, 11 g protein, 7 g fat (4 g sat), 127 g carbs, 340 mg sodium, 149 mg calcium, 15 g fiber

references

Chapter 1

Craig WJ, Mangels R. Position of the American Dietetic Association: vegetarian diets. *J Am Diet Assoc.* 2009;109(7):1266–1282.

Rastogi S et al. Why do patients with heart failure suffer from erectile dysfunction? *Int J Impot Res.* 2005;(17):S25–S36.

Dissanayake D et al. Effects of zinc supplementation on sexual behavior of male rats. *J Hum Reprod Sci.* 2009 Jul;2(2):57–61.

Schneider R et al. Stress reduction in the secondary prevention of cardiovascular disease. *Circ Cardiovasc Qual Outcomes.* 2012;(5):750–758.

Lutz A et al. Regulation of the neural circuitry of emotion by compassion meditation: effects of meditative expertise. *PLoS ONE.* 2008;3(3):e1897.

Digby J. What does sperm smell like? Does it smell bad? LoyalMD. [Internet]. 2017 Sept 1. Available from: https://www.loyalmd.com/what-does-sperm-smell-like/

Ferrari ND et al. Smelling like dead fish: a case of trimethylaminuria in an adolescent. *Clin Pediatr (Phila).* 2006 Nov;45(9):864–6.

Chapter 2

Yamada T et al. Erectile dysfunction and cardiovascular events in diabetic men: a meta-analysis of observational studies. *PLoS One.* 2012;7(9):e43673.

Inman BA et al. A population-based, longitudinal study of erectile dysfunction and future coronary artery disease. *Mayo Clin Proc.* 2009 Feb;84(2):108–13.

Nehra A et. al. The Princeton III consensus recommendations for the management of erectile dysfunction and cardiovascular disease. *Mayo Clin Proc.* 2012 Aug;87(8):766–778.

Chapter 3

Cassidy C, et al. Dietary flavonoid intake and incidence of erectile dysfunction. *Am J Clin Nutr.* doi: 10.3945/ajcn.115.122010.

Maiorino MI, et al. Effects of Mediterranean diet on sexual function in people with newly diagnosed type 2 diabetes: the MED-ITA trial. *J Diabetes Complications.* 2016 Nov-Dec;30(8):1519–1524.

Havlicek J, Lenochova P. The effect of meat consumption on body odor attractiveness. *Chem Senses.* 2006 Oct;31(8):747–52.

Pill-free ways to improve your sex life: exercise, smoking cessation, and alcohol moderation can help bring sexual activity back into the bedroom. *Harv Health Lett.* 2014 Aug;39(10):4.

Hall, S et al. Sexual activity, erectile dysfunction, and incident cardiovascular events. *Am J Cardiol.* 2010 Jan 15;105(2):192–7.

Smith G et al. Sex and death: are they related? Findings from the Caerphilly Cohort Study. *BMJ.* 1997 Dec 20–27;315(7123):1641–4.

Wright H et al. Frequent sexual activity predicts specific cognitive abilities in older adults. *J Gerontol B Psychol Sci Soc Sci.* 2017 Jun 21.

Yang H et al. Does serum homocysteine explain the connection between sexual frequency and cardiovascular risk? *J Sex Med.* 2017 Jul;14(7):910–917.

Dabbs J and Mohammed S. Male and female salivary testosterone concentrations before and after sexual activity. *Physiol Behav.* 1992 Jul;52(1):195–7.

Steinke EE. Sexual dysfunction in women with cardiovascular disease: what do we know? *J Cardiovasc Nurs.* 2010 Mar-Apr;25(2):151–8.

Leitzmann M et al. Ejaculation frequency and subsequent risk of prostate cancer. *JAMA.* 2004;291(13):1578–1586.

Chapter 4

Radnitz C et al. Investigation of lifestyle choices of individuals following a vegan diet for health and ethical reasons. *Appetite.* 2015 July;90:31–36.

Eisenberg M. Testosterone replacement therapy and prostate cancer incidence. *World J Mens Health.* 2015 Dec;33(3):125–129.

Chapter 5

Olweus D et al. Circulating testosterone levels and aggression in adolescent males: a causal analysis. *Psychosom Med.* 1988;(50):261–272.

Twenge J et al. Sexual inactivity during young adulthood is more common among U.S. millennials and iGen: age, period, and cohort effects on having no sexual partners after age 18. *Arch Sex Behav.* doi: 10.1007/s10508-016-0798-z.

Chapter 6

Beezhold B, Johnston C. Restriction of meat, fish, and poultry in omnivores improves mood: a pilot randomized controlled trial. *Nutr J.* 2012 Feb 14;(11):9.

Chapter 7

Haub MD et al. Effect of protein source on resistive-training-induced changes in body composition and muscle size in older men. *Am J Clin Nutr.* 2002 Sep;76(3):511–7.

Zenico T et al. Subjective effects of Lepidium meyenii (maca) extract on well-being and sexual performances in patients with mild erectile dysfunction: a randomised, double-blind clinical trial. *Andrologia.* 2009 Apr;41(2):95–9.

Akhtari E et al. Tribulus terrestris for treatment of sexual dysfunction in women: randomized double-blind placebo-controlled study. *Daru.* 2014 Apr 28;(22):40.

Punyawudho B et al. A randomized, double-blind, placebo-controlled crossover study of Cappra for the treatment of mild or mild to moderate erectile dysfunction in Thai male. *Afr J Tradit Complement Altern Med.* 2012 Dec 31;10(2):310–5.

Ito TY et al. The enhancement of female sexual function with ArginMax, a nutritional supplement, among women differing in menopausal status. *J Sex Marital Ther.* 2006 Oct-Dec;32(5):369–78.

Gianfrilli D et al. Propionyl-L-carnitine, L-arginine and niacin in sexual medicine: a nutraceutical approach to erectile dysfunction. *Andrologia.* 2012 May;44 Suppl1:600–4.

Gliozzi M et al. Bergamot polyphenolic fraction enhances rosuvastatin-induced effect on LDL-cholesterol, LOX-1 expression and protein kinase B phosphorylation in patients with hyperlipidemia. *Int J Cardiol.* 2013 Dec 10;170(2):140–5.

Mollace V et al. Hypolipemic and hypoglycaemic activity of bergamot polyphenols: from animal models to human studies. *Fitoterapia.* 2011 Apr;82(3):309–16.

Mollace V et al. Bergamot polyphenolic fraction counteracts erectile dysfunction occurring in patients suffering from type 2 diabetes. *PharmaNutrition.* 2016;(4):S41–S46.

Mahajan GK et al. Efficacy of aphrodisiac plants towards improvement in semen quality and motility in infertile males. *J Complement Integr Med.* 2012 Feb 17;(9):Article 6.

Thu HE et al. Eurycoma longifolia as a potential adoptogen of male sexual health: a systematic review on clinical studies. *Chin J Nat Med.* 2017 Jan;15(1):71–80.

Kotirum S et al. Efficacy of tongkat ali (Eurycoma longifolia) on erectile function improvement: systematic review and meta-analysis of randomized controlled trials. *Complement Ther Med.* 2015 Oct;23(5):693–8.

Chapter 8

Crowe B. The effects of yoga participation on symptoms associated with menopause: a mixed methods study. [PhD thesis]. [Clemson (SC)]: Clemson University, 2013. 250 p.

Chapter 9

Meeker J et al. Phthalates and other additives in plastics: human exposure and associated health outcomes. *Philos Trans R Soc Lond B Biol Sci.* 2009 Jul 27;364(1526):2097–2113.

Biesanz Z. Dildos, artificial vaginas, and phthalates: how toxic sex toys illustrate a broader problem for consumer protection. 25 *Law & Ineq.* 2007;25(1):203.

resources
FOR VEGAN SINGLES AND COUPLES

by Ellen Jaffe Jones

FINDING YOUR VEGAN SOUL MATE

If finding a vegan soul mate is where your heart is headed, here are some resources to help you in that search. As I've mentioned earlier, traditional in-person dating services or speed-dating meetings often don't include any criteria for matching dietary preferences. Online dating services have been around for a long time and also provide varying degrees of success. There's nothing quite like meeting people for the first time in real life versus meeting them after you've fallen for a creative version of themselves on a dating site.

Vegan meetups are often a way to get to know single vegans in your area. At first you might feel intimidated walking into a crowded restaurant or someone's home and not knowing anyone, but everyone there is in the same boat, so dive right in. Meetups are usually free and often are set up as potlucks. The organizers may request that each dish be accompanied by a written recipe or list of ingredients to accommodate anyone with food sensitivities.

To find some of the possible vegan meetups happening around the world, go to meetup.com/topics/vegan. Vegan festivals often sponsor meetups around the date of the event. To get a list of festivals in your area, go to vegan.com/festivals.

Here are some specific resources if you're in the market for a vegan date. These listings are always changing and evolving, so search under "resources for vegan singles and couples" to get both local and distant options.

Elite Singles: elitesingles.com

Although this site doesn't cater exclusively to vegans or vegetarians, it's vegan friendly.

Green Singles: greensingles.com

Not specifically vegan but very vegan friendly.

My Vegetarian Dating: myvegetariandating.com

Registration is free but access to more extensive services and to communicate with other members requires a fee-based subscription.

Veg Love (formerly Veg Speed Date): findveglove.com

Organizes events in different cities where participants can have mini-chats and socialize with prospective partners who share common vegan concerns.

Vegan Dating: vegandating.org

Registration is free but access to more extensive services and to communicate with other members requires a fee-based subscription.

Vegetarian Dating Service: vegetariandatingservice.com

Setting up a profile and browsing are free, but access to the full extent of services requires a fee-based subscription.

Vegetarian Passions: vegetarianpassions.com

It's free to set up a profile, browse, and connect through social media. Upgraded memberships are available for webcam chats.

VeggieConnection.com

A site for vegetarians, vegans, raw foodists, and fruitarians seeking romance and friendship. You can set up a profile and search for free, but contacting members has different levels of pricing.

VeggieDate: veggiedate.org

Members include vegans, lacto-vegetarians, ovo-vegetarians, pescatarians (fish-and-vegetable eaters), semi-vegetarians, and others who are working toward a vegetarian or vegan lifestyle. Profile setup is free.

VEGAN CONDOMS AND LUBRICANTS

Vegan is so mainstream now that you can search any online store, even ones that aren't exclusively vegan, and discover dozens or even hundreds of vegan options.

Condoms

Vegan condoms are becoming increasingly numerous and available, and companies are adding vegan options to their lines to meet consumer demand. Most of these options are not only vegan but are also free of the spermicides and chemicals typically used on nonvegan condoms. Information on popular brands can be found at the following online sites:

B Condoms: bcondoms.com

Fair Squared: fairsquared.info

FC2: fc2femalecondom.com (latex-free female condoms)

Glyde: glydeamerica.com

L.: thisisl.com/collections/shop

Sir Richard's: sirrichards.com/condoms

Sustain Natural: sustainnatural.com/products/condoms

Lubricants

Almost Naked Personal Lubricant: goodcleanlove.com

Astroglide Natural Feel Liquid: astroglide.com

Sliquid: sliquid.com *(all products are vegan and some are organic; also sells Buck Angel's T-Lube for trans men)*

VEGAN SEX SHOPS

Online retailers often come and go or reinvent themselves. You'll find a current list of vegan retailers at afemmecock.com. Here are a few of the best-known ones:

Etsy: etsy.com

A popular source for a wide variety of handmade and vintage items, including vegan sex products made by small businesses.

The Frugal Domme: frugaldomme.com

Offers a large selection of BDSM products hard to find on other sites.

SheVibe: shevibe.com

Everything you could want in sex toys, clothing, and BDSM products. Not only promotes vegan clothing but also features a top-of-the-line phthalate-free dildo that's waterproof, splashproof, and rechargeable. It has ten modes and, of course, "comes" with an app.

Smitten Kitten: smittenkittenonline.com

Fun place that stocks tons of vegan products with cute names. Be sure to check out Nipple Nibblers Tingle Balm and let me know how that works out for you.

The Vegan Sex Shop: thevegansexshop.com

Sells condoms, candles, and all kinds of sex toys, with one of the largest selections of all-vegan sex items on the web. Six percent of profits go toward the animal rights or human rights charity of your choice.

index

Recipe titles appear in *italics*.